Toxicology!
Because What You Don't Know Can Kill You

Alan H.B. Wu, Ph.D.

lh

Sa Francis, CA

Feb 2016

Toxicology! Because What You Don't Know Can Kill You contains fictitious characters, events, and places. Any resemblance to actual persons, living or dead, business establishments, events, or locales is entirely coincidental. The science described in these stories, however, is factual.

ISBN-13: 978-0-989-3485-1-5
eBook ISBN: 978-0-9893485-0-8

Dedication

This book is dedicated to my wife Pam, who believed that these stories needed to be told, my daughter Kim for her artwork, editing, and marketing, my son Edward for the website design (www.alanhbwu.com), and my son Marcus for his review of these stories.

Table of Contents

Prologue

We all wish we had more power. The power to turn back time, to re-write history and make better decisions, but most importantly, the power to save a life. However, the dream of being someone's hero or even saving yourself from certain death or misfortune, is a plight that no average person can seemingly muster. Without super strength or extrasensory perceptions, it may appear that we are on our own to battle uncertain destiny. But what if I were to tell you there's more? There's a way to change your fate, to hold more cards, and take not only your own life, but the lives of those you love into your hands. No, we cannot go back in time, but we can set forth ripples of change into the future that can alter our coexistence forever. Toxicology and clinical laboratory testing may be one of those portals.

Clinical toxicology is a branch of medicine dealing with human poisonings and poisons. These doctors have the responsibility of bringing patients who are poisoned back to health. A major part of clinical toxicology is the analysis of blood, urine and other body fluids to determine what the intoxicants are and how much is present. For the past 30 years, I worked as a professor of laboratory medicine and director of a toxicology laboratory. The goals of my laboratory's investigations were to find the best therapeutic management of patients and to uncover if poisoning was the cause of death.

Part of my job as director is also to defend the results of clinical laboratory test results in criminal and civil courts. This involves reviewing data and medical files, and giving depositions and court testimonies. Often these lawyers need my expertise to interpret results of toxicological testing.

This book is a compilation of stories based on my involvement in court cases over the past 30 years. The characters depicted in the stories are fictional. Any similarity to any actual person living or dead is coincidental and unintentional. However, the scientific information and court proceedings presented are accurate and based on real cases.

Max's Quiet-a-Time

****

Max was not a particularly endearing or loving man, but he provided well for his family. He did not drink heavily, and always came home to his wife each night. Although he attended most of his kids' soccer games and swimming meets, he often had one eye on the clock and one foot out the door. By the time he reached his 70s, his wife had died, and two of his daughters moved out of the area. Only Gail, the youngest, stayed in town and would occasionally come by the house to see her Pop.

Gail was shy and reserved. She had a string of boyfriends but none of them stayed around. Gail held a steady job as a law clerk. Because she never married, she was devoted to her father. When his health started to fail, she took over his affairs. It was Gail's decision to put Max into an assisted living facility when he fell and broke his hip, and then into a nursing home a few years later when he began forgetting things. Shady Elm, with its advertised "peace and tranquility for all residents in their golden years," seemed to Gail to be the perfect place for Max. But these decisions were hard on her because she had to make them alone. Her sisters were too busy with their own lives. They provided some money but little else in the way of the emotional support that Gail really needed.

After two years in the nursing home, Max was nearly eighty, and his health began to deteriorate rapidly. He used to be a large man with a healthy appetite, but he started losing weight due to the bland food at the home. Gail could see that her father started giving up on life. His mind began fading. He would have short bouts of anger and outrage followed by long periods of deep depression. The staff at Shady Elm began to resent him and would look forward to giving him his daily dose of quetiapine. This drug is used to treat schizophrenia and bipolar disorder, neither of which Max ever suffered from. Nevertheless, it appeared to help Max get through some of his difficult moments. In the nursing log, caregivers noted each day when it was Max's "quiet-a-time."

Visiting on what was to be Max's last Saturday, Gail noticed a significant change in her father. He was shaking uncontrollably and had a high fever. She begged the nurses to send for the doctors, but the head nurse said that it was the flu that was going around the unit and there was nothing more they could do that night. By Monday morning, Max was dead. The doctors at Shady Elm signed out the death as due to "old age" and denied Gail's request for an autopsy.

Undaunted, Gail arranged for Max's body to be sent out for a private autopsy. The pathologist's report noted moderate atherosclerosis of the heart but without acute occlusions, mild muscle atrophy, and advanced arthritis. In other words, Max had the heart and joints of an old man, but these were not the cause of his death. The pathologist ordered toxicology tests on the postmortem blood. The report revealed a higher than normal level of quetiapine in his blood. Max had indeed been on quetiapine, but the result was higher than expected. Nevertheless, the pathologist was unable to conclude if this was

2

the cause of Max's death.

A voracious reader and internet surfer, Gail spent the next several months learning about quetiapine and its side effects. Her sisters wanted her to stop investigating and move on with her life, but their comments only made her more committed. She was convinced that there had been some foul play but she didn't know how to prove it. Gail wasn't as interested in pursuing legal action as she was in finding the truth and gaining closure over her father's death.

Gail remembered that her boss at the law firm once hired me to help them on a wrongful death lawsuit. A few months after Max's funeral she went into her office, found my business card, and called. She told me that her father died at a nursing home and that she was suspicious that his death might not have been from natural causes.

"I have the pharmacy records from the nursing home and the autopsy report," she said. "I'd like for you to review these and see if you agree with the pathologist's conclusion of a natural death. Dad was an angry man at the end and I think the nurses just wanted to keep him calm. And by the way, Dad's nursing notes from his last weekend at Shady Elm are missing."

Never one to back down to a challenge, I replied, "Send me the PDFs, Gail. But I make no promises that I'll find anything different from the conclusions rendered by your pathologist."

When I received the documents from Gail, I immediately went to the final toxicology report. The decedent's postmortem quetiapine blood level was high at 952 mcg/mL; the therapeutic concentration in living people is between 100 and

500 mcg/mL. Dr. Lisa Beaumont, a former student of mine, was the pathologist who signed out the case as "death by natural causes." Lisa was drop-dead gorgeous and had all the other residents pining for her when she was in training. She was a little twisted though, because while all the others just wanted to sign out biopsies, she asked for autopsies so she could dig into the corpses.

I called Lisa now and asked, "Why wasn't the high quetiapine level considered in the manner of death in this case?"

Lisa replied, "It was you who first taught me about the phenomenon of postmortem redistribution." After death, blood levels can artificially increase to several-fold higher levels than at the time of death due to leakage from neighboring tissues. The extent of seepage depends on the condition of the body and the time interval between death and the autopsy. Lisa continued, "After discussing this case with our forensic toxicologist, we decided that although the quetiapine level was higher than therapeutic, we took into account the redistribution phenomenon in issuing our report. We tend to be very conservative; you can appreciate this in the litigious society of ours."

Not looking for more work, I normally would have accepted this explanation. But there was something about this case that didn't feel right; maybe it was the missing nursing records or the pain I'd heard in Gail's voice. So I dug further.

Under my advice, an attorney at Gail's office issued a subpoena to the pathology office requesting the "toxicology litigation package" from Max's case. This is the original data and printouts from the equipment used in testing Max's blood. The

4

final report was prepared from calculations made from these documents. When I received the data, I found that Lisa's lab used gas chromatography/mass spectrometry, state-of-the-art analytical equipment for forensic toxicology. I could not find any fault with the performance of the test or the calculation of the result. I was relieved that my former student's conclusions were sound and defensible, but at the same time, felt disappointed for Gail. I was about ready to give up when I noticed on the last sheet of reports, as an incidental finding, that prochlorperazine was also found in Max's blood. Lisa had ignored this finding because toxicology labs do not normally test for this drug as it is not particularly toxic. There was a small peak in the printout indicating that the drug was present, but no concentration was computed. Could this result help me prove that postmortem redistribution had *not* occurred for quetiapine and that, instead, Max died of an overdose of the drug?

I quickly called Gail to ask about her father's medication. She said that he had been given both quetiapine and prochlorperazine. Shady Elm's pharmacy records showed that standard dosages were prescribed for both drugs for the past 12 months. I then called my former student to ask if any blood specimens remained from Max's autopsy. The pathology lab's policy was to only retain samples for six months unless special provisions were made so save them, and Max's autopsy had been 8 months ago.

"We would be up to our vitreous humor if we kept all specimens for longer than this," Lisa said. In her crazy world of death investigations, I knew that she meant they would be up to their eyeballs. Then I asked Lisa for a favor: to run one more analysis.

"I don't know how that will help," she said, "but I'll get the lab techs on it." The following week, my requested analysis was printing out on my fax machine. I anxiously scoured the lines on each page even before it completed printing. On the last page, I found what I was looking for. There was also a hand scribbled note from Lisa: "You owe me for this—the next brew is on you."

Remembering Lisa's stunning figure, I said to myself *I'm there.*

I called Gail and said, "Call your lawyer; we're going to sue Shady Elm."

Following months of discussion, a deposition was finally scheduled on the case of the descendants of Max Lewis v. Shady Elm Nursing Home. Present were Gail and her attorney; the defense attorney for Shady Elm, George Stencil; a court reporter; and me, the one being deposed. After preliminary questions about my qualifications, Stencil got right to the meat of the deposition.

"Doctor, even your hired pathologist listed the cause of death as 'natural.' You were not even at the autopsy, correct?" I nodded but Stencil told me he needed a verbal response. I obliged. Confidently, Stencil went on, "How can you then state that the cause of death was quetiapine toxicity?"

I replied, "The pathologists did find a toxic level of this drug but discounted the finding because of postmortem redistribution," and went on to explain what that meant. "However, I have some new data that refutes this notion." This was the new data I had received from my former student.

Stencil, in a rather bold and confident voice: "But my sources said that the tox lab didn't have any more samples for you to test. So how can you have any new data?"

Me: "From the pharmacy records at Shady Elm, the decedent had been given daily dosages of both quetiapine and prochlorperazine as antipsychotic agents. From the lab findings after death, only the quetiapine was high. If postmortem redistribution took place, both drugs would have been high."

Stencil: "But the lab didn't have a level on prochlorperazine, so how could you conclude this?"

Me: "Eight months after Max's autopsy, I had the lab calibrate the same instrument that was used in Max's blood testing using fresh prochlorperazine standards. This enables us to get an estimate of this drug's concentration."

Stencil: "But the lab didn't calibrate its reading for prochlorperazine when Max's autopsy was performed. How can you conclude these levels are accurate now?"

Me: "The equipment used then is the same as today. The retention time shows me that the testing drug condition was also the same. The 'chromatographic retention time,' which every drug has, is the time interval from when the sample is injected into the instrument to when a peak appears." Pulling charts out to clarify, I continued, "As you can see, the retention times at 5.15 minutes for prochlorperazine is unchanged from 8 months ago when the decedent's blood was tested. By comparing peak area from Max's blood to the calibration recently produced, I calculated a blood level that fell within the expected therapeutic range for this drug. It was not in the toxic range."

Stencil: "And this means what? "

Me: "If there was postmortem redistribution, both the prochlorperazine and quetiapine would be high. The fact that only quetiapine concentration was high told me that it was at toxic levels before his death."

Stencil started back pedaling: "Is this procedure of 'historic calibration' within established forensic standards?"

Me: "Some labs do use calibrations established a few days or weeks ago. The use of historic calibrations dating back 8 months admittedly is not standard practice. However, I can state that it is more likely than not to be accurate, which is the standard for civil lawsuits such as this."

Stencil paused for a few minutes, and then said in a modulated voice: "I have no further questions for you." Under his breath he said, "We'll see about this."

Two weeks later, Gail called me with news of the lawsuit. "After your appearance, we deposed one of the nurses in my father's care on the evening before his death. We told the nurse that the pathologist changed the cause of death to quetiapine overdose based on your deposition. When we asked her to recount the events of that evening she said that my father was really agitated and was disturbing the sleep of the other residents. The charge nurse said to give him a double dose of quetiapine in hopes of calming him down. Apparently they had been doing that for several days prior to his death and it always worked. Being new to the unit, the evening nurse was reluctant to deliver the dose, but she did not want to go against her supervisor. She made a note in my father's nursing record to cover herself for this action. She was then told that those notes had been lost and were not available for verification of her action. At that point, she

looked at me and my lawyer and began sobbing. I could sense
that she was blaming herself for my father's death. With no more
questions, she rushed out of the law office where the deposition
was being held. When we deposed the head nurse, she denied
ordering extra quetiapine for my father. Nevertheless, Shady Elm
terminated her employment and settled the case with us before
closing arguments. We never found out who destroyed the
nursing records but we all suspected that it was the head nurse."

I asked Gail, "How did your sisters react to this
outcome?"

"My sisters all of a sudden became interested in me, or I
guess, in the large settlement award. I told them that they didn't
deserve any. Maybe that was little harsh, but I didn't care. But my
lawyers said that they were entitled, so we're going to split the
settlement equally."

That night Gail climbed into bed and let out a sigh of
relief. She smiled knowing that she did the right thing for her
father. She gained a new confidence in herself and vowed that
from that point forward, her life would be different. She
reconciled with her sisters. They were the only family she had
left. When they were in town, they would all visit Max's grave
together and say a prayer. Gail soon left the law firm and
enrolled in law school. She knew that nothing could be more
challenging than what she went through with her father's case.
She met a fellow law student and they moved in together. "This
time," she said to herself, "this one is here to stay."

*

*Anti-psychotic drugs such as quietiapine are dangerous and must only be
given with the appropriate medical indications. There is a great*

variability of response from person to person. Once it has been determined that these drugs are helpful for a given patient, their continued usage must be carefully supervised by qualified physicians. Nurses are more aware of changes in a patient's day-to-day behavior, and can be trained on how to look for evidence of drug toxicity. It is ironic that anti-psychotic drugs that themselves are highly toxic are given to patients who are unstable and potentially suicidal. Doctors are providing the means for their own patient's demise. I have hope that my discovery of the pharmacology abuse in Max's death may lead to legislative reform regarding the oversight of nursing home practices. Though this will require changes in the law and will take time, I have personal reasons for this hope: it won't be long before my fellow baby boomers and I become recipients of dependent care.

Second Chance

****

Joan Cain was a child of the 60's. Her given name was Candice, but she hated it because the kids in school used to call her "candy cane" and "candy bar." When she was sixteen, she legally changed to Joan, after her favorite folk singer, Joan Baez. When she was seventeen, in the summer of 1969, she hitchhiked from her home in Oneida, New York to the Woodstock festival to hear Baez sing. Her parents were divorced and her mother drank heavily, and didn't care about her. Soon after she'd gone to Woodstock, Joan left home altogether and hitchhiked her way to California. She had ten dollars in her pocket. Eventually, she moved in with some new friends, all long-haired hippies. During that time, she drank just like her mother had, smoked a lot of pot, freebased cocaine, took acid, and occasionally shot up with heroin. She worked at odd jobs—waitressing, pressing clothes at a dry cleaner, caretaking at a nursing home.

When Joan was in her early thirties, she was in a traffic accident. She broke several ribs from hitting her chest on the steering wheel and suffered facial damage from the windshield. Back then, there were no air bags in cars or laws for seatbelt use. Joan was hospitalized for several months. While she'd never been beautiful, she had an attractive smile; after the accident, she was disfigured from facial scars. Her injuries also caused her chronic pain and she was told that she would have to be on pain medication for the rest of her life. She continued her drug abuse and five years later contracted non-A, non-B hepatitis from an infected syringe. Medical virologists later isolated this virus and it was renamed hepatitis C.

By the time she was forty, Joan had enough and decided to clean up her life. She went to school to become a physical therapist. She stopped her drug and alcohol abuse, and cut her hair short. Nobody from her high school days would recognize her now.

Unfortunately, her hepatitis did not spontaneously resolve like it did for some patients. Her disease had entered the chronic phase, and was eating away at her liver. By age 59, Joan was in fulminant hepatic failure. She became jaundiced, the sclera of her eyes turned yellow, and her skin began itching as a result of high bilirubin, a bile pigment that was responsible for her coloration. She also had excess ascites fluid in her abdomen. Joan checked into the University Hospital where Dr. Bloom, a liver specialist, told her she needed a liver transplant.

Jeffrey Bloom was a compassionate physician dedicated to his patients. Although he wasn't old, in this regard he was from the old school. He made it a point to answer all questions his patients and their families about their medical care. The medical practice he belonged to had recently been transferred to a health maintenance organization. He was getting increasing pressure from his practice administrators to see more and more patients and spend less time with each. He absolutely hated what they were asking of him, but he realized that he had to comply with their demands in order to remain competitive.

When Dr. Bloom saw Joan, he assessed whether or not she was an appropriate candidate for a liver transplant. There was a long waiting list for qualified individuals, as the demand for organs greatly exceeded the supply. Joan's chronic hepatitis C infection did not disqualify her for the transplant. However, her previous drug and alcohol use was a concern for the surgical team. Joan provided documentation from her employer and personal doctor that she had stopped using drugs and alcohol more than ten years ago. She was now a model citizen and deserved serious consideration. As part of the organ screening process, Joan underwent a standard urine drug test. The results came out negative for alcohol, marijuana, and cocaine—the vices of her youth. It came as a shock, however, when she was told that her urine was positive for amphetamine-like drugs.

Joan was confused; she never used methamphetamine or Ecstasy. As was within her rights, she requested a repeat urine drug test, hoping that there had been some mix-up in the laboratory; but the repeat result was again positive. Joan pleaded with Dr. Bloom to investigate, insisting that there was something wrong with the test. Believing Joan and hoping that there was a reasonable explanation, Dr. Bloom called me regarding Joan's test result.

I explained to Dr. Bloom that two tests were conducted on each of Joan's urine samples: "The amphetamine screening test is sensitive for amphetamine, methamphetamine, and Ecstasy. We also perform a confirmatory test based on mass spectrometry. Although her urine was devoid of these three drugs, we found that a designer amine was present in her urine." Dr. Bloom had heard about these drugs but wanted clarification.

I continued, "Internet chemists are now operating out of home labs to produce new chemicals that have similar physiologic properties to illicit drugs. They are termed 'designer' because some clever chemist has altered the drug's structure while maintaining its physiologic effect. In this case, we found a mass spectral match for one of the more popular designer drugs we've been seeing among our patient population recently."

Bloom asked, "Could some of the other medication that Joan took have been responsible for the false amine result?"

"Send me the medication list and we'll check the literature and specifications on the package insert of the assays," I responded.

Dr. Bloom called Joan and asked her what prescription and over-the-counter drugs she was taking. Like many people of her age, Joan was on several medications. She replied, "Lipitor for my heart, Synthroid for my thyroid, sometimes zolpidem to help me sleep at night and some drug that starts with a 'T' to relieve my chronic pain."

"Tylenol?" asked Dr. Bloom, to which Joan replied, "Yes that's the one."

Armed with this information, I went back to my office to see if any of these drugs had been reported to interfere with the amphetamine assay. I wasn't hopeful of finding anything, because these were common medications and we would have known by now if there was an interference with these drugs and our tests. Although the news was not good for Joan, I was relieved when we found no interference, and I called Dr. Bloom to tell him.

Dr. Bloom informed Joan of my conclusion. "There was

14

no error, and the lab stands by their test," he reported. "I am sorry to say, but at this point, we are forced to remove your name from the active liver transplant list. We have other medications for your chronic hepatitis that will keep you comfortable but it won't cure your liver. We'll let you know if the situation regarding a transplant should change."

Confused and dejected, Joan left the office. She was so upset that she could not formulate any words. She resigned herself to the fact that she would probably die soon. Without the transplant, Dr. Bloom gave her six months, maybe one more year.

She sat alone in her car in the parking lot and wept. "I've lived my life irresponsibly. I have no family, I've made no contributions to society, and I've made no one's life better. It's time for me to atone for the decisions I've made in my life." She turned on the ignition and drove home. In her remaining days, she had to put her financial affairs in order. She wanted to leave her assets to a physical therapy foundation.

I went about my business without thinking much more about Joan's case. I had heard denials of drug use by patients and didn't believe most of them. Joan in particular had a lot to gain by not admitting to drug abuse. I knew that although drug-screening tests were flawed, we had definitive, confirmatory results by mass spectrometry. I was a little bothered initially by the fact that the patient was older and didn't fit the demographic profile of designer amine abuse. But these days, nothing surprised me as to what people will do to themselves. At the time, I was preoccupied with the lecture that I was giving at a conference the next month as an invited speaker.

My talk at the conference was on bath salts. These were designer amines that recently flooded the market. They were a new type of recreational stimulant labeled as bath salts in order to confuse law enforcement, parents, and teachers. Packets were available under names like Ivory Wave, Hurricane Charley, and Vanilla Sky. These drugs were popular because they were easy to get, and they produced a buzz similar to methamphetamine and cocaine. Also important was the fact that they weren't detected by conventional drug-screening methods. Our testing methods for drugs-of-abuse are not perfect. They can't detect some recreational drugs, while other legitimate prescription drugs produce a positive result for recreational drugs.

After my lecture, I wandered around the poster exhibits to see what was new. These exhibitions were often given by students and young scientists in the field. Abstracts are submitted to the meeting organizers, reviewed by a scientific committee, and selected authors are invited to present their work at the meeting in the form of a display. During the poster presentation itself, presenters are required to stand next to the poster and answer any questions that conference attendees might have about their work. It's an important opportunity for young investigators to network with other scientists who have the same research interest.

In the last row, I spotted one poster that particularly piqued my interest. It was a pharmacology paper on the human metabolism of a lesser used analgesic drug. I thought to myself, *Hmm, maybe Joan was telling the truth when she denied amphetamine use. There may be an explanation for her positive drug test result after all.* When I arrived back at the office, I had one of Joan's original urine sample retrieved from the freezer and ordered it to be checked for trazodone. We learned years ago that it was prudent to save urine samples that are positive for one drug or another. While it took up a lot of freezer space, these saved samples had become useful on numerous occasions. At first, the lab couldn't find the drug I was looking for in the urine. Another unknown substance was present that was blocking the instrument's ability to see trazodone. I ordered the sample to be re-tested using a different set of extraction conditions. The second time around, we found the drug we were looking for. *I may have been wrong in not believing Joan*, I thought.

I immediately called Dr. Bloom to discuss Joan's case. Without telling him what I suspected, I asked Dr. Bloom to re-check the drugs that Joan was taking. In the past, I have told doctors that when asking for a medication history, self-reporting by patients is often unreliable. Many drugs sound alike and patients are often confused as to what medications they are on. I wanted an independent verification of my findings. Dr. Bloom did not have Joan's original pharmacy records as he was not her primary physician. Bloom also didn't want to raise Joan's hopes by contacting her directly. So instead, Dr. Bloom placed a call to Joan's personal doctor in order to get her prescription records. Dr. Bloom then remembered that Joan said a drug starting with a "T".

He called me right away. "We discovered that Joan is on trazodone, not Tylenol as we previously thought. But how does that help her case?"

It was then that I told Dr. Bloom what I had learned at the conference. One of the posters outlined the chemical structures of trazodone and its various metabolites. Since I'd just reviewed studies on designer drugs for my lecture, I recognized that there was a trazodone metabolite, *m*-chlorphenyl piperazine, that has a similar structure to methamphetamine. When I got back to the lab, we re-tested Joan's original sample and found trazodone and its metabolites. No one before had shown that trazodone could interfere with the amphetamine test. As a final confirmation, I personally took a trazodone pill. After four hours, my urine tested positive for the designer amine due to the presence of this metabolite.

Bloom asked, "So what does this mean for Joan?"

I said, "We believe that she did not abuse a designer amine. You should reconsider putting her back on the transplant list."

Dr. Bloom deeply regretted that he didn't have all of the right information prior to his decision on Joan's case. Now that he knew that Joan did qualify for a liver transplant, he hoped it wasn't too late. He called up the United Network of Organ Sharing, a non-profit organization that manages the organ transplant system in the United States. They added Joan's name to the list of recipients needing a liver. Dr. Bloom requested that her name be back-dated to their original request because of the mistakes he made in the case, and because Joan's situation was becoming dire.

In the meantime, Joan changed her life. To the extent that her health permitted, she became a volunteer at a local shelter for the homeless, serving food and providing emotional support.

After 18 months on the list, Joan was still 71 patients away from a liver donation. Some patients jumped ahead of her because they'd had unusual tissue types that were good matches with a particular donor. A good tissue match reduces the chances of organ rejection by the recipient, the leading cause of transplant failure. Even with good matches, however, recipients must take "immunosuppressant" drugs that block their white cells from attacking the new organ. Sometimes the drugs themselves produce toxicities if given at the wrong dosages, so blood must be tested at regular intervals to determine if the drug concentration is within the accepted therapeutic range.

Unfortunately, Joan never got to that stage. She passed away while still on the transplant list. Her primary care physician informed Dr. Bloom of Joan's death so he was able to attend her funeral. This is the worst part of my job, Dr. Bloom thought to himself. Sure, Joan made mistakes in her life. But she'd turned things around and she deserved a second chance.

*

There are over 84,000 men and women on the active transplant list in the United States. Most livers are harvested from otherwise healthy individuals who have unexpectedly died, such as after motorcycle crashes. In 1992, California enacted the Helmet Law for motorcyclists. While this decreased deaths by 37%, it also reduced the number of available organs for transplantation. This shortage has led to reports of criminal harvesting of organs from live un-consenting patients, particularly for kidneys, as an individual can survive with only one.

Individuals wishing to donate their organs after their death can indicate this wish on their driver's license. The "opt in" option is used in most countries. In some countries, such as Spain, there is an "opt out" option. In these countries, your organs will be taken after death unless you specifically indicate otherwise, which has made organs more readily available in these places. Some individuals refuse to indicate organ donation upon death because they fear premature termination of a life support system. Others have religious reasons for not donating. Therefore, organ donation will never be mandated. In most cases, ignorance is the reason people don't list themselves as organ donors. Only when a family member or friend needs an organ donation does the topic typically get discussed.

Like Joan Cain, many will die before a suitable donor becomes available. But there is hope. Medical scientists and biomedical engineers are working on creating human organs through stem cells. Under proper stimulation, these cells, derived from embryonic or fetal tissues, have the ability to differentiate into mature cells that function just like the native ones found in the organ. Although this research is still many years, or even a decade away from being ready to be implemented, it is hoped that laboratory-produced organs may be able to alleviate organ shortages worldwide.

Blood Beer Making

Ever since grade school, Joel Miller and Teddy Norris had been the best of friends. They lived a few blocks apart in a neighborhood of predominantly working-class people. They were both from broken families. Joel's father left his mother when he was five years old and Teddy's parents were divorced when he was nine. Joel was an only child and lived in a trailer with his mom. His mother died when Joel was 22. Teddy lived in a low-income apartment complex with his mother and younger sister. Teddy's uncle also lived in the apartment. He was an alcoholic and would verbally abuse him when he was drunk. Both moms worked long hours in order to make ends meet. This left a lot of idle time for the two boys during the day. Knowing this, several rival gangs tried to enlist Joel and Teddy. But they stuck together and resisted the temptations. This often led to threats, bullying and some beat downs by gang members, but nothing serious ever happened. Other than a little mischievousness of their own, the two boys were largely good kids. Joel was big for his age. He began shaving when he was 13, and by the time he was 17, he looked like a young adult. He had no problem getting beer and wine at the local liquor store. Back then, they didn't check IDs as rigorously as they do today. Joel and Teddy used to go down to the riverbank to skip rocks, talk about girls, and drink beer.

Neither Joel nor Teddy had the inclination or financial means to go to college. They were also adverse to the idea of joining the military. So after finishing high school, they got odd jobs in the area: painting, yard work, gas station attendant, pizza delivery. They met every week or so at the local saloon to drink their troubles away. Joel was the heavier drinker. While a six pack of beer was sufficient in the beginning, he gradually needed more to satisfy his alcohol cravings. By the time he was in his late twenties, he had progressed to hard liquor because it got him loaded faster. Teddy saw that Joel was becoming an alcoholic and tried to get him to stop or at least slow down. When Joel refused, he started seeing less and less of his old friend. Joel was in denial about his drinking problem. He convinced himself that he could handle the alcohol and that it didn't affect his work. He got a steady job as a night janitor at a nearby corporate office. Other than the night watchman, there was no supervision at night. So he often came to work inebriated.

As long as I do a good job cleaning, he said to himself, *I can drink and work at this forever.* Since he wasn't married and his living expenses were minimal, his work was more than sufficient to finance his only hobby, drinking.

Teddy settled down and got married. He met his wife at a party at a friend's house. At the time, Teddy was unemployed. So he and his wife moved downstate to be closer to her family. Teddy found a job as a driver for an express package delivery company. Within five years, he and his wife had two young children. Teddy got along with his mother-in-law, who often came over to help with the kids. Teddy only drank occasionally and never more than a few glasses of wine. Unlike in his younger days, he never got drunk anymore. As a driver, he was regularly tested for drugs and alcohol. With a family to support, he didn't want to risk losing his job.

Joel, on the other hand, began losing control of his alcohol use. On the way to work one night after a binge-drinking episode, he was stopped by the police for swerving off the road. The police asked him to step out of the car, and they conducted a field sobriety test. He was asked to walk a straight line and to count down backwards starting at 100. He was unable to accomplish either. They asked him to blow into a breathalyzer, which registered an alcohol value of 0.18%, more than twice the legal driving limit. Based on this reading, Joel was issued a DUI and sent to jail, where he remained for four days. With his one call, he contacted his boss and told him he was sick with the flu.

"You don't want me to infect the offices while I am cleaning, do you?" he said. His boss agreed and told him to stay home. Joel was fined $1000. His driving license was going to be suspended for six months, but he argued that he needed to drive to work each day, so he was granted a restricted license. He could drive to and from work, but only on the specific days and coinciding with his work schedule. He also had to complete the state's DUI Program.

Joel was able to curtail his heavy drinking to just the weekends and days off from work. He couldn't stop drinking altogether. His license was fully restored after six months. Shortly thereafter, he began his former heavy drinking habits again. Joel didn't have a support system for long-lasting rehabilitation. He had little in his life — no family, no girlfriend, his best friend Teddy moved away, and nobody at work to talk to.

It was only a matter of time before he would be charged with a DUI again. When that happened, he spent 90 days in jail and was fined another $1000. He also lost his janitorial job. They told him they would lay him off so that he would be eligible for unemployment benefits. His life was spiraling out of control.

Desperate to turn his life around, he turned to religion. He found a priest who recognized his plight and took him in. Father O'Neil was the minister of the St. Francis church for nearly 30 years. He had seen many people like Joel. In exchange for a room in the basement of the church, Joel performed different jobs in and around the church. Sometimes it involved grave digging on church grounds, which he didn't mind. He had been at the church for a few months when a mutual friend of his and Teddy's from the old days recognized Joel and asked if he was going to their 15-year high school reunion.

"I heard that Teddy was coming," he told Joel. It had been six years since Joel last saw his childhood friend. Excited at the prospect of seeing Teddy again, Joel called the alumni group and told them he would be coming to the reunion.

When the date arrived, Joel arrived at the school, clean and sober. He hadn't had a drink since joining the church. He saw Teddy and they hugged. Teddy was a little heavier but otherwise he looked the same. They reminisced about old times. When the reunion was over, Joel asked Teddy to join him for a drink at the old tavern they used to go to. Teddy drank a little more than normal because he was happy to see his old friend.

Joel could not resist the temptation to drink either. Joel could always handle alcohol better than Teddy. Although he did have several drinks, he didn't think he was actually drunk. Just after the call for last drinks at the bar, Joel told Teddy that he would take the wheel of Teddy's rental and drive them both to Teddy's hotel. Teddy told Joel that he could stay in his hotel room that night, rather than going back to the church. Teddy didn't know that Joel had his license suspended because of two prior DUIs. But he was in no position to argue.

As they drove into the dark and rainy night, it was just after 2:00 a.m. Father O'Neil would be giving his service in six hours and Joel was supposed to be there to open the church. There were only a few other cars on the road, but Joel was not able to see well or judge the speed of the rental car, which was a hybrid and didn't produce any engine noise.

Joel didn't intend to speed, but it had been a while since he'd driven a car, and was surprised about how different this one was. He took a turn too slowly and the car slid off the road. He jammed on the brakes, which made the car slide even more. The passenger side of the car collided sideways against a large oak tree. There was no side air bag in the car. The impact from hitting the tree trunk caused the passenger door and window to smash into Teddy's head, and his body slumped toward the driver's side of the car. Teddy was unconscious and his head was bleeding profusely.

Joel was dazed but largely uninjured. It would be several minutes before he was able to climb out of the car. He didn't have a cell phone and didn't know where Teddy's phone was. He stumbled to the road and within a few minutes saw the headlights of a car. He stood in the middle of the road and waved his hands for the car to stop. When it did, two teenage boys got out and saw what happened. They called 9-1-1. Firemen arrived within a few minutes. Teddy's legs were trapped underneath the wreckage. The firemen brought in the Jaws of Life to extricate Teddy from the car. It took 30 minutes before they could get him out. An ambulance and paramedics were waiting at the scene. When his body was freed, they strapped him onto a gurney and rushed him to the hospital. He had a massive head injury. He was not breathing and the paramedics could find no pulse. They did CPR and chest compressions in the ambulance. Unfortunately, by the time he arrived at the hospital, Teddy was dead.

Joel was also sent to the hospital for his minor wounds. The triage nurse noticed a distinct odor of alcohol and she noted this on the nursing notes of his medical record. Blood was collected, paperwork signed, put into an evidence bag and sealed. It would be sent to the city's toxicology lab. The ED staff kept Joel overnight and released him the next morning. Waiting for him in the discharge area were two uniformed officers. They arrested him on a charge of drunk driving and operating a motor vehicle with a suspended license. It was his third offense. He was taken to jail. Later, he was charged with vehicular manslaughter for the death of his friend Teddy.

Joel did not get permission from the jailhouse to attend Teddy's funeral. He imagined that there would be a lot of crying from his family and angry words spoken about Joel. It was best that he couldn't attend. The district attorney, Malcolm Adams, reviewed Joel's file and history of DUI arrests. Given that he was driving without a license and that he killed his passenger while intoxicated, he changed the charge from manslaughter to second degree murder. He was determined to get a long prison sentence so that Joel could not endanger anyone else in the community.

At the arraignment, bail was set at $500,000. Since Joel was not employed and had no income or savings, he remained in prison. He had no place to go anyway.

Although Teddy and Joel were taken to my hospital, I didn't learn about this accident until the DA contacted me. Victims of alcohol-related traffic accidents were common at the General. I was asked to comment on Joel's blood alcohol reading taken from the emergency department and tested in the county's forensic lab.

On the charge of second degree murder, Joel Miller was defended by Jefferson Brown, an African-American lawyer just two years removed from passing the bar exam. He had taken a job at the county's public defender's office. Since Joel had no money to hire his own lawyer, Jefferson was assigned to the case.

"Everybody thinks he's guilty," he said to Sherry Lane, a first-year law clerk assigned to him. "I want you to find out how errors can be made in blood alcohol tests," he told Sherry. Jefferson thought that if he could get Joel acquitted, it would gain him some positive notice, and possibly open some doors for him to move up. But he had to provide convincing arguments in order for him to win the case. The clerk came back after two weeks all proud of herself and said just three words to Jefferson relating to Joel's case.

"In vivo fermentation," she said.

"Say that again?" was Jefferson's reply.

"I found a case report in the literature, where a diabetic patient with a yeast infection in his bladder, produced ethanol as a byproduct of fermentation," Sherry explained. It's the same process that is used to make beer. You need an enzyme — that's supplied by the yeast; then you need a substrate — that's the blood sugar; and you need an oxygen source — that's in the air. Then voilà, alcohol! Okay, I know it's a little far-fetched, but in reviewing Joel's medical records, he did have high glucose. So he needs to say that it stings when he pees. You know, like in a urinary yeast infection. We women get that all the time."

Jefferson sat back and thought for a moment. "This is not so far-fetched, my young friend. We know he was drinking, but was he legally drunk? His blood alcohol from the crime lab was 0.145%. Because it was sent over the weekend, the testing was conducted 3 days after blood was taken. If part of his alcohol production was due to in vivo fermentation, it might put him just below the limit. "

The wheels were turning in both Sherry's and Jefferson's heads. "We need to get a microbiologist who will say in court that this could happen," Jefferson said.

He hired a retired microbiologist who was an expert witness "for hire." The public defender's office had some funds for expert witnesses. Give them a plausible hypothesis and they will defend it, for a fee and a large one at that. Jefferson asked the court to rule on the admissibility of the ethanol data on Joel Miller. If this data was excluded from the case, it would be difficult to prove that Joel was drunk at the time of the accident. The arguments were put in front of the judge in the absence of the jury. Jefferson put the "expert" microbiologist on the stand, and he calmly concluded that there was no way to rule out in vivo fermentation as a partial cause of the alcohol reading in Joel's blood.

Now DA Adams had a difficult task at hand. He had to

absolutely refute the notion raised by the defense counsel. He asked me about these opinions rendered by the defense.

I testified. "Indeed, in vivo fermentation, that is, production of ethanol within the body itself, could occur, but usually in the context of postmortem cases. Bacteria invade dead bodies as part of the putrification process.

Jefferson then asked, "Doctor, what about *in vitro* fermentation?"

I responded, "In vitro fermentation is the production of ethanol within the test tube after blood collection. It can occur if there is prolonged storage of the blood at increased ambient temperatures."

Jefferson continued. "There was a delay in the testing of Mr. Miller's blood by the crime lab. If I told you that the specimen had been sitting in a hot police car for several hours, would that change your opinion?"

I replied, "Ah, but I have evidence from the medical record that Mr. Miller's blood was positive for ethanol at the time of ED admission." This came as a shock to the defense attorney.

Jefferson asked, "Is this new evidence? Was this disclosed earlier? Did the DA know about this?"

I answered no to all questions. "I was not asked this question until just now when you asked it."

I went on to explain, "As part of our routine testing, we performed a serum osmolality. This is a measure of undissolved solutes in blood. The normal constituents of osmolality are the electrolytes, glucose, and urea. We have a formula that accurately predicts the serum osmolality from these measured parameters. When the formula result doesn't match the measured osmolality, this suggests the presence of a low molecular weight drug found at high molar concentrations. Ethyl alcohol is one of those constituents. Since Mr. Miller did have a difference between measured and calculated osmolality, the ethanol concentration at the time of emergency admission exactly accounts for this gap. Because this testing was done immediately after blood was drawn, there is no possibility of in vitro fermentation."

Jefferson called for a recess and consulted with his microbiologist for hire. Not being an enzyme chemist, he had no reply. The judge presiding over the case ruled that the ethanol data was admissible. The trial began and the jury learned of Joel's previous DUI arrests. This was his third strike. They also heard that he was legally drunk and drove on a suspended license when he caused the accident that killed his friend. The DA portrayed a reckless person whose alcohol addiction consumed him. He was a menace to the public. The jury agreed. Joel Miller was convicted of second degree murder. His sentencing hearing would be determined separately. Malcolm Adams thanked me, as I'd saved the case with my disclosure. We were both glad that Joel Miller would not be out anytime soon.

Joel Miller was sentenced to 15 years in prison. He was a model prisoner and served 10 years before he was paroled. He never drank again. He went back to the church where Father O'Neil was waiting. He took him in and never asked Joel anything about the circumstances of the accident.

*

The claim for in vivo fermentation with regard to blood alcohol testing has never been upheld in civil or criminal court when testing is conducted on a stat basis by a clinical laboratory. This is despite the fact that thousands of DUI cases are litigated each year. This case was an example of an egregious misinterpretation of scientific principles, disguised as expert testimony, in order to sway a legal opinion.

There have been reports of in vitro fermentation. In one case, urine samples from patients who have a documented yeast infection and diabetes were sent through the mail to a drug-testing laboratory. The urine arrived four days later, having been transported at room temperature. This is a "perfect storm," where there was a fermenting enzyme present (yeast), a substrate (glucose), sufficient incubation time, and sufficient temperature for the fermentation reaction to take place. However, the amount of alcohol produced, even under optimum conditions, is small compared to the amount seen in DUI cases.

Serum osmolality testing is available at almost every hospital in the country. It is used to detect toxic alcohols, such as methanol and ethylene glycol, and not to support ethyl alcohol testing. Therefore results of osmolality testing are not usually available.

Urine Luck

****

In high school there are the preppies, the jocks, the drama queens, the nerds, and the potheads. Jaco was clearly in the last category. He spent much time in the bathroom smoking cigarettes or an occasional joint before attending class. "I'm never going to need to know this shit," he told his mother. His mother knew that he wasn't dumb, just unmotivated. His car reeked of cigarette and marijuana smoke. Butts and crumpled rolling papers crammed the dashboard ashtray. He kept his windows closed for fear that the smell would reveal him to the school narcs, but everyone knew what he was up to anyway and didn't care.

Jaco was always good with cars and motorcycles. The kids brought all their mechanical problems to him. So when Jaco left high school, his classmates were not surprised that he was able to land a steady job as a garage man at the city's bus depot. By then, he was smoking dope regularly, but it didn't interfere with his job. He became a master at concealing his drug use from his superiors. He worked at the bus depot garage for eight years and they eventually transferred him to driving the city's bus. This was easier than working on engines. The promotion, however, required him as with other drivers, to undergo routine urine drug and alcohol testing.

Jaco did not want to lose his new job by failing a urine

test; he needed the money to support his drug lifestyle. He was able to stop smoking hash for a month while he started his new job. In the meantime, he learned all he could about drug testing policies and procedures so he could beat them. If he had studied this much in high school, he could have been a lawyer by now. One of the first things he found out was that you can buy at-home urine drug-testing kits on the Internet. These tests were similar to the lab-based test his employer used. Although purchasing these kits on a regular basis got expensive, it was better than losing his job with a positive drug test. The bus company scheduled their drug test quarterly. Since they did not do them randomly, his plan was to abstain from smoking five days prior to the appointment. He tested his own urine using the kit just to be sure.

"If I test positive, I'll just call in sick that day," he told his unemployed co-druggie roommate. This plan worked for several years. But he wanted more. He believed he could beat the test without even having to stop smoking before the test.

Why should I cease my enjoyment four times a year? he thought. His new plan was to drink copious amounts of water to dilute his urine just prior to self-testing. Jaco learned that in order for his urine to come out positive, the amount of drug in the urine had to exceed the test's threshold. He got this down to a science; he knew exactly how much he could smoke and how much water he needed to drink to get below the test cutoff. Besides, he always owned the 'I am sick today' excuse as his get out-of-jail card. This worked for years. He knew he was playing with fire, but he couldn't get off pot.

*

Calvin was in the nerd set in high school. His parents emigrated from Taiwan when he was two years old. He did well in math and made friends through the science club. He was small for his age having reached puberty later than the other boys. He was shy around girls at school; most of them were bigger than he was. While they went to the same school, Jaco and Calvin didn't know each other. Their only encounter was when Calvin was a freshman and Jaco was in his fifth year of high school. Calvin desperately had to pee before algebra. Not knowing the unofficial bathroom rules, he went into the smoker's john. Jaco and his friends saw the little kid, pushed him against a stall, and told Calvin to beat it. After that encounter, Calvin said to himself, *someday I'm going to stand up to those guys.*

Calvin went to college, majoring in chemistry. Science was easy for him, and he was eager to learn. Right out of college, he got a job in my toxicology laboratory. We were doing workplace drug testing at the time. Calvin's job was to process the hundreds of urine samples each day and load them into the instruments for testing. He felt overqualified for this work, but he had to start somewhere. The worst part of the job was the awful smell. Sometimes, he would spill some urine onto his clothes, shoes, and socks. Fortunately we had a shower in the lab and he kept extra clothes on hand. I recognized that Calvin had a keen eye for details, and I wanted him to advance.

After a few years, I asked Calvin, "Why don't you go back to school and earn your master's degree in forensic science, which includes those involved with workplace drug testing? Then we can have you do more interesting jobs that suit your talents." With that encouragement, Calvin enrolled in night school while keeping his day job working for me. When Calvin finished two years later, I promoted him to certifying scientist. His new job was to look at toxicology data and verify their results. By now, he was no longer the shy introverted person he'd been when he was young. Calvin met a girl, got married, and together they had a daughter named Jenny.

*

Jaco's urine sample was routinely sent to the lab for testing. Unknowingly, Calvin had been involved with Jaco's urine testing for years. The samples were identified by number only. Jaco's samples were simply labeled as #32449. In going through his daily records, Calvin noticed that one sample reported as negative was just below the cutoff for THC. THC is tetrahydrocannabinol, the active ingredient of marijuana. This sample also contained a low level of creatinine. While creatinine is a normal component of urine, low values indicate urine dilution by higher than normal fluid intake. Calvin went back into the records and found that #32449 consistently produced these results. He came to my office to show me what he had discovered.

I told him, "Some people have other drugs or constituents in their urine that may trigger a false reaction to the THC test. Our cutoffs differentiate between what is truly positive from interferrents. Besides, people can have small amounts of marijuana in their urine due to passive exposure. Calvin, you wouldn't want us to report a positive result just because someone was at a rock concert and exposed to others who were smoking, would you?"

"I guess not," he said. But Calvin wasn't satisfied. How

36

could #32449 be at a rock concert each time he was drug tested? Although he knew he could get in trouble for this, Calvin kept one of #32449's urine samples aside in the freezer. He removed it one day when I was away. Opening the cup, he let it stand at room temperature to let some of the water evaporate. When this concentrated urine was retested, it came out positive. *I've got my eye on you #32449*, he said to himself, and then discarded the cup.

Jaco's driving record was without incident. This eventually landed him a job driving kids at his old high school. They were mostly freshmen and sophomores who didn't have drivers' licenses yet or whose parents couldn't afford cars for them. He was ten years older than most of them and they treated him like he was Fonzie from Happy Days; the cool driver dude. He still had to undergo regular drug testing and he still was participant #32449. By this time, he'd gotten tired of drinking excess fluids prior to his tests and learned about adulteration products. He purchased Urine Luck from the Internet in hopes of taking his deception to the next level. Urine Luck was a commercially available urine drug-testing adulterant. It consisted of a vial containing one ounce of a yellow fluid. It arrived through the mail in an unmarked package. The user was instructed to add the liquid in the vial to a urine sample while in the privacy of the bathroom before submitting the specimen to the urine collector. Urine Luck oxidized drugs to other compounds, thereby producing a false negative urine drug test result. Jaco tried it out with his at-home drug-testing kit and found that it worked for marijuana. By this time, he also began experimenting with heroin. Urine Luck worked on this drug too. Jaco went online and purchased enough of the adulterant to last him for three years of quarterly drug testing.

Back in the lab, Calvin noticed something was now different about #32449's urine. His previous urine samples were odorless and colorless, a reflection of his dilute urine. Now, this sample was not near the threshold value, and had a much deeper yellow color. The creatinine level was also now within normal limits. Calvin thought that maybe #32449 had reformed and was now clean. But then he thought, *I don't buy it. He's doing something else.* On a whim, and totally against the rules, Calvin took a solution of THC and added it to one of #32449's samples that previously tested negative. To his astonishment, the repeated test remained negative, even though the added THC should have produced a positive result.

He is definitely doing something again, Calvin thought. *In order to solve this problem, I have to think like a drug user trying to hide my addiction. What would I do if he were me?* Calvin knew that subjects who are drug tested urinate in the privacy of a bathroom without a witness. Maybe #32499 was adding some chemical to invalidate his test. So he went on Google and typed in "adulteration and urine drug testing." There was a hit for Urine Luck. After reading about how this adulterant worked, Calvin came straight to my office. "Do we have permission to test suspicious urine samples for the presence of adulterants such as this?" he asked, showing me the Internet article. I emphatically replied, "We can't do that today. Taking that sort of action would be viewed as a witch hunt. But I'm part of a group of other toxicologists who are trying to get the regulations changed so that we *can* do this type of testing. For now, though, we have to be careful that we don't single anyone out." With that Calvin bit his tongue and went back to his office.

About two years later, fervor about adulteration practices did lead to changes in the federal drug testing policy. Labs were mandated to check for evidence of adulterants. The new law required testing of all urine samples, not just the suspicious ones. A positive adulterant result was worse for the participant than a positive drug test, because it amounted to fraud. The lab developed tests for adulterants, including Urine Luck.

Calvin couldn't wait until #32449's urine showed up in the lab again. Meanwhile, Jaco had gotten wind of these rule changes. He knew he had to stop using Urine Luck. "Now what am I going to do?" he asked his roommate. The stakes were higher. He'd stopped using marijuana and was instead using heroin regularly now. Like most addicts, he had to have a hit almost daily and could not quit. He had also become the driver for the elementary school children. Unbeknownst to Calvin, his own daughter, Jenny, was one of Jaco's daily passengers.

Two months after the new drug testing regulation was in force, the results of #32449's urine appeared on Calvin's desk. It was positive for morphine, the heroin metabolite.

"We finally got him," Calvin said to me that day. "Now maybe he can be prosecuted accordingly."

I replied, "This is his first offense. He'll have an opportunity to defend himself. This is not over yet."

Jaco met with a medical review officer, or MRO. He explained that he'd had a clean toxicology record for ten years, and that this was all a big mistake. Jaco had seen a Seinfeld episode and remembered that Elaine had a positive urine result due to poppy seed ingestion, which contains morphine. He remarked in an innocent tone to the MRO, "I ate a poppy seed bagel yesterday. Could that have had any effect?"

The MRO responded, "Yes, poppy seeds are well known to contain morphine. I'm going to recommend that the bus company put you on probation. From now on you'll have to submit to monthly drug tests and they'll be randomly scheduled. We will also arrange to have someone witness you urinating into a cup. You better clean up your act buddy. Real fast."

Hearing the outcome of the MRO's hearing on #32449 and that he was only on probation, Calvin was livid. He became obsessed with trying to prove that #32449 was a drug addict. After a few days of research, he came across an article in a toxicology journal by researchers at the University of Connecticut. The investigators showed that testing urine for the presence of thebaine could be used to confirm poppy seed ingestion. Thebaine is not present in street heroin as it is not derived from the poppy plant. Excited, Calvin showed me the article and asked if the lab could test #32449's urine for thebaine.

"No Calvin," I replied. "You're getting too personally involved in this one case. If you don't drop this, you may face disciplinary action." But Calvin disobeyed. He did set up a test for thebaine and examined #32449's urine without my knowledge or permission. As he'd suspected, the result was negative, indicating that #32449 was lying about his positive test result.

I knew it, damn it, he said to himself. *He is a drug user.*

The next week, Jaco went to work driving the school bus. He had just taken a hit of heroin. It was a rainy day, and his vision was impaired. It didn't help that he was also in an opiate haze. He swerved across the center line and hit a woman and a child in their car head on. The children on the bus were thrown about. There were no seat belts. There were loud screams followed by crying. Miraculously, neither he nor any of the children on the bus were seriously hurt. The driver and passenger of the car, however, both died at the scene, their car crushed by the oncoming speeding bus.

Calvin heard the news on the radio and was horrified. The bus was carrying kids from Jenny's school. A chill ran down his spine. He frantically ran to his office to grab his cell phone to call home. Then he remembered that his wife had taken Jenny to the dentist and that Jenny was going to miss school. She was not on that bus. A crowd in the lab gathered in the break room where the news was being reported on local television. The station interrupted the regularly scheduled daytime soaps. A few minutes later, Calvin's cell phone, which was still in his hands, unexpectedly rang. It was from the police.

*

Testing for adulterants by forensic laboratories continues to evolve and improve in order to catch cheaters of the drug-testing system. Unfortunately, "garage" chemists also evolve by developing new adulterating agents that are designed to mask positive urine drug test results, while escaping detection of their use. Moreover, adulteration testing countermeasures add to the cost of testing the drugs themselves.

I believe there is a good deal of hypocrisy surrounding the federal workplace drug testing laws in the U.S. today. On the one hand, drug use while working has its penalties. On the other, it is legal in many states for manufacturers to produce products purposely designed to allow someone to pass a drug test. The scope of testing is also incomplete. For example, the mandated testing for phencyclidine, or Angel Dust, makes little sense when the prevalence of this drug is so low. Meanwhile, the abuse of many other drugs, like oxycodone, goes on unabated. I realize that testing for a wide panel of drugs is impractical and costly. But improvements in testing policy must be made.

Why did the police call Calvin? Re-read the last two paragraphs again.

Sloe Gin

****

All emergency departments in the U.S. see their share of alcohol-related hospital admissions, as this drug is highly toxic. High consumption can be fatal in some individuals, particularly teenagers and young adults who binge drink and are new to alcohol use and abuse. In a hospital, patients often present with altered mental status. It is often not possible to determine if a patient's medical condition is due to too much alcohol consumed, the presence of some other drug, or some other medical reasons. Alcohol use is also a factor for trauma patients who have been involved in a motor vehicle accident. My clinical laboratory is responsible for testing blood alcohol levels in our patients. Most of these patients recover in the morning, after their levels have subsided. Alcohol testing in a hospital is not typically performed for law enforcement purposes. Nevertheless, test results can be subpoenaed by attorneys and results used in criminal cases and civil lawsuits. I have frequently been asked to render interpretations of alcohol test results in court or via a deposition.

These legal cases are nuisances to us as they sometimes ask our technologists to appear in court. They are questioned as to whether or not they followed procedures that day with regards to alcohol testing. Since we do thousands of tests every day, it is impossible for anyone to remember any one particular test. So I agree to appear to discuss our policies and procedures, and if I can render some interpretation of results, both the court and my laboratory are better served.

There are three commonly asked questions that are posed to toxicologists in court. 1) "If someone drinks a specified amount of alcohol, what will his peak alcohol concentration be?" To answer this question, we need to know how big the person is, how much alcohol the individual consumed and over what period of time. Typically, one beer is equal to a glass of wine and a shot of whiskey. 2) "If the blood alcohol level was 0.10% at the time of testing, what was it two hours earlier, e.g., at the time of a traffic accident." Once all of the alcohol has been absorbed into the blood, it breaks down at a rate of about 0.015 to 0.020% per hour, so this is a simple calculation. 3) "Was the person impaired at the time of the event or accident?" This is the most difficult question, because impairment occurs at different alcohol concentrations depending on the individual's genetics and prior alcohol experience. An experienced drinker can handle much more booze than a naïve one.

*

In the case of Olivia Schaefer, all of these issues and others were raised to me as an expert witness. Dr. Schaefer was an obstetrician and gynecologist and was a junior member of a group practice. One day after a three-day weekend, she arrived at her office and was described as "a little out of sorts" by her senior colleagues. Like many ob/gyn practices, their group had their share of malpractice lawsuits regarding deliveries of babies that resulted in some unexpectedly poor medical outcomes. While their rate of complications was below the national average, nevertheless, these types of lawsuits against obstetricians are common. The head of the practice, Dr. Graham Heater questioned Dr. Schaefer about her alcohol use.

"I drank three glasses of wine at dinner last night but none since" was Dr. Schaefer's response.

Dr. Heater responded, "Olivia, you know how much our program is scrutinized by our malpractice insurance carrier. Our rates are sky high. Just to be on the safe side, I have to administer a breath alcohol test on you before you begin your day."

"I have nothing to hide, please proceed" was Dr. Schaefer's response.

One of the ultrasound technicians trained in administering the breath alcohol test was called. In the privacy of an empty exam room, Olivia was asked to blow into the device. After a minute, the result read "0.035%."

"There must be some mistake. I had nothing to drink today. Can we repeat the test?"

"Did you use mouthwash today?" The tech asked.

"Yes, like I always do each morning" Olivia responded.

"Our policy is to wait 15 minutes before a repeat test is given. In this way, any recent mouthwash will have dissipated" the tech said.

Olivia was asked to wait in the break room and asked to not consume any beverages during this time. Her appointments were covered by other members of the group. When the repeat test produced essentially the same result, Dr. Heater was notified.

"Olivia, our insurance mandates that we institute a zero tolerance policy regarding alcohol use. Anyone over 0.02% must be suspended and your results reported to the State Medical

Board." Every state has a medical board empowered to protect patients from incompetent or compromised physicians by revoking medical licenses.

"I am afraid I have to send you home. You will be given an opportunity to discuss your case with an independent Medical Review Officer that we have a contract with. They may suspend your medical license or put you on probation. Please don't say anything at this time. You might want to contact your lawyer."

In tears, Dr. Schaefer left the office and went home. After she calmed down, she contacted her attorney, Mr. Frank Kimball, and explained her situation.

*

Frank responded: "Once your license has been revoked, it is very difficult to get reinstated. If you really didn't have any alcohol for 24 hours, you may be one of the rare individuals who are a slow drug metabolizer. These individuals have a deficiency in the liver enzyme that breaks down alcohol in the body. We can test you to see if you are one of these people" Frank told Olivia. "I know an analytical toxicologist at the General Hospital who can help us."

I had worked with Frank before and found him to be a very competent attorney. Frank prided himself for having a better than average grasp of medical science and he was a chemistry major in college. When Frank called, I was happy to work with him again. Once fully briefed, I suggested that we perform a human controlled experiment with Dr. Schaefer. We arranged for her to come to my office at noon just after drinking three glasses of wine over a one hour time period. This was not considered research, but rather a medico-legal issue, so permission from ethics committee was unnecessary. When she arrived, I arranged to have an intensive care nurse on hand to install an intravenous "heparin lock" into the arm of Dr. Schaefer, where it was kept for the remainder of the afternoon. This enabled us to draw blood from her at hourly intervals without having to insert a needle into her each time blood was needed. Dr. Schaefer was told to not consume any other alcohol, food or beverages during this interval. Five blood samples were collected starting at 1 pm and ending at 6 pm. Each of these samples was tested for alcohol in my lab. Her first sample produced an alcohol reading of 0.065%. Subsequently, her blood alcohol declined at a rate of just 0.003% per hour. This was one fifth of the normal rate.

"So she is a slow metabolizer!" I said to my lab tech.

He quickly responded, "How do we know if she was drinking just a little to keep her alcohol content in her body from declining?"

"This is possible" I responded, while thinking that this was a very astute comment on my tech's part. "I think it would be very difficult to titrate her alcohol intake to match a constant metabolic rate over 5 samples" I commented. "We saw a very steady rate of decline. If she was also drinking, the metabolic rate might be more variable over time."

Satisfied that Dr. Schaefer was a slow metabolizer, I called Frank and informed him of my conclusion.

"You will be pleased to know that Dr. Schaefer does have an exceptionally slow rate of alcohol metabolism." I then gave him all of our data. "If she indeed only drank 3 glasses of wine in the previous night in question, the results from our little study show that she could still be positive the next morning." But then I cautioned Frank, "This might not get her off the hook with the medical board which states that no licensed health care workers should have any measurable alcohol content in their blood while attending to patients. We might still have to argue that she was not impaired by this low amount of ethanol but her claim of not drinking on the job may be proven by this study."

Frank was very pleased with the results and called Dr. Schaefer with the good news. Having served on medical licensing boards myself, I believed that the board would give her probation and allow her to keep her license. Alcohol consumption is not prohibited and many doctors have beer or wine with their meals the night before seeing patients. At Dr. Schaefer's hearing, she was reinstated with a stipulation that no alcohol could be consumed by the doctor for at least 48 hours prior to seeing patients. The board warned her that in the future, a positive alcohol test result while on the job would result in license revocation irrespective as to when it was consumed. Dr. Heater further warned Olivia that alcohol testing on her will be conducted if there is a complaint by a patient or if there is an unexpected outcome due to a procedure that she performed.

*

I didn't think much of Dr. Schaefer's case again until a few months later when a patient came into our emergency department following consumption of methanol. Unlike ethanol, small amounts of methanol can cause blindness and death if not treated immediately. Methanol is found in automobile windshield wiper fluid and other sources and is sometimes consumed by alcoholics and homeless people when a source of ethanol is not readily available. The toxic effect of methanol occurs following its metabolism to formaldehyde and formic acid. One way to treat methanol poisoning is to administer fomepizole, a drug that blocks methanol metabolism by the liver enzyme alcohol dehydrogenase, the same enzyme used to break down ethyl alcohol. The methanol poisoned patient was treated with fomepizole resulting in his full recovery.

It was this case that led me to ponder if Dr. Schaefer had taken some fomepizole in order to retard her rate of ethanol metabolism prior to consuming alcohol for our study. She might not really be a slow metabolizer and was drinking on the morning that she had a positive result. Since my laboratory performs unknown toxicology analysis in blood and urine, we have the capability of looking for fomepizole in the blood of Dr. Schaefer. All of her samples were still in my freezer. I quickly called Frank, explained my suspicions, and asked for permission to test Olivia's blood for this drug. I did not get the answer I was looking for.

"I was hired by Dr. Schaefer to get her license reinstated. We have accomplished this task. I have no obligations to reopen this issue."

"Do you know if Dr. Schaefer has access to fompeizole or even know about this drug?" I asked. "This is not a court trial but a licensing hearing." I pleaded. "Can you ask her if she took any drugs before she came into my lab for the study?"

"Even if I ask, you know that I have client-attorney privileges and cannot disclose any communications between her and me. No law has been broken so I am not obligated to recuse myself."

I continued to plead this issue with him: "But if she is not a slow metabolizer, she may be drinking on the job. In that case, she may be jeopardizing the health and safety of her patients."

"Under no circumstances are you allowed to test her samples. I am sending over a courier today to pick up the remaining amount of serum you have on her."

This situation was a dilemma for me and my lab. I immediately called the attorneys at the General Hospital and explained that this is a medical safety issue. They stated that I had no real evidence to suggest that Dr. Schaefer was cheating. Therefore the existing medical privacy laws superseded our desire to know the truth even if some patient's health was at stake. I was forced to relinquish her remaining samples to the courier and was told that the samples would be promptly destroyed.

*

Kathie Bradie was a 16-year old girl who was dating her older brother's friend. She really liked the boy but he kept pressuring her for sex. Because she was a virgin, she was reluctant. One Friday night, she gave in because their relationship had reached the point that she sensed that if she continued to refuse him, he would break off their three-month relationship. Kathie insisted that he used a condom. Unfortunately, the condom failed and Kathie became pregnant by him. Against the wishes of her family, she sought an abortion very early during her pregnancy and went to see Dr. Olivia Schaefer. Olivia was out late with her boyfriend the previous night and was drinking until 2:00 am. When she came to work at 8:00, Kathie was her first appointment. Olivia did a good job of hiding her symptoms from the nurses and colleagues, but she had a terrible headache, was dizzy and nauseous. Nevertheless, she performed the abortion on Kathie.

The procedure did not go smoothly. Kathie bled excessively

and was hospitalized. Dr. Heater became aware of the situation and Dr. Schaefer was tested again for alcohol. When the result was 0.035%, he contacted the Medical Board who promptly revoked her medical license. Soon after the hearing, Dr. Heater discharged Dr. Schaefer from their medical practice.

I was sick to my stomach when I heard about this situation. Kathie's injuries could have been avoided if I had made my suspicions known to the Medical Board. In retrospect, I should have insisted to her attorney that we had the right to examine the blood sample for signs of adulteration before I agreed to conduct this experiment of ours. It was fortunate that Kathie's bleeding episode was not serious and she recovered without any further medical incidence.

With this case, my professional relationship with Frank Kimball as an attorney ended. While I understood that his primary objective was to protect his client, I held him partially responsible for Kathie's injuries. He never called me again for any other alcohol-related cases.

*

Methanol and ethylene glycol poisoning are infrequent but not rare. They tend to occur during the winter months when homeless patients need something "to take the chill away." These toxic alcohols lower the freezing point of water and enable these subjects to tolerate the cold. Fomepizole has been shown to be highly effective in treating patients who consume these toxic alcohols. The drug was approved by the FDA under the Orphan Drug Act. This act enables a quicker and less expensive path for drug approval because the disease that fomepizole treats is uncommon and the expenses to do a full trial for FDA drug clearance would be prohibitive. The alternative and much more inexpensive treatment regimen is to administer ethyl alcohol intravenously. Ethyl alcohol also slows down the conversion rate of methanol and ethylene glycol as it competes with alcohol dehydrogenase. It is ironic that a patient consumes methanol because they want to get drunk and ethyl alcohol is not available. When they arrive to the emergency department, they are given the ethanol that they need to survive and the goal of being alcohol intoxicated is achieved.

Alcohol and drug abuse continues to be a major problem among health care workers. Physicians in particular know the negative health consequence of alcoholism. Despite the high stakes involved with the revocation of a medical license, many physicians cannot resist the temptation to imbibe. As such, many will go to great lengths to hide their addiction. Dr. Schaefer's claim and possible cover-up of fomepizole was particularly insidious if true. It is not clear how Dr. Schaefer might have known about fomepizole as she is neither a toxicologist nor pharmacologist. But I found out later that she did a year of residency in emergency medicine before switching to obstetrics and gynecology and must have learned about fomepizole then. She may have gotten some drug from a former colleague. Dr. Schaefer entered a drug rehabilitation program and hopes to practice medicine again one day.

Country Doctor

****

Dr. Rupert Ford was the community doctor for Red Plains, California for the past 55 years. Dr. Ford was born in the late 1920s, when Red Plains, originally a mining town, consisted of just 500 people. Over time, the population grew to about 2,000 residents, but it was still largely a small, agricultural town. Everybody knew each other and each other's business. Eventually, Rupert Ford became known as "Doc Ford" or just plain "Doc." Considering how small Red Plains was, the town considered themselves fortunate to have their own doctor; town residents did not have to travel to get primary medical care. Doc delivered or was involved with the delivery of many of Red Plains' residents. For some of the long-time residents, he had delivered four generations of babies. Although Doc Ford was now in his early eighties, his mind was still very sharp and he remained a skilled diagnostician.

He told his patients, "I don't need most of that fancy dancy medical equipment that younger doctors need. I rely on these hands, ears, and eyes, and the stuff between these ears."

For the most part, Doc Ford was right. With his stethoscope, he could detect the slightest murmur of the heart or crackling sound of the lung. His fingers had the feel for the smallest lumps or protrusions as early signs of cancer. Other doctors who trained with Doc Ford as general practice physicians were amazed at what a good physical exam and basic laboratory tests could reveal in the hands and mind of the right person. One of the best things about Doc Ford was his medical judgment. He knew when there were serious conditions requiring more advanced medical treatment. He would refer these patients to the "big city" doctors. When patients did not have serious illnesses, he would tell them to just go home and rest.

"Remove your stresses and let the body heal itself," he would say as a big believer in holistic medicine. "Eat right, get plenty of rest and exercise, and clear your mind of unnecessary clutter," he would tell his patients. "As much as possible, you should stay away from that hooch." That was probably his best advice.

Doc Ford had a small office in the middle of town, with one receptionist, Priscilla, and one nurse, Betty Johnston. Betty had been with Doc Ford for over 25 years. Priscilla was her oldest daughter and had just started working for Doc within the last two years. Years ago when he was first starting out, Doc had his patients pay him in cash or in credit at their store if they owned a place of business. These days, however, he was obligated to go through the usual insurance channels for reimbursement for his services. Occasionally, he would make a house call if it was for somebody who didn't have a car and couldn't travel to the office. To keep his medical skills sharp, Dr. Ford would spend a few days each month in the emergency department of the Collinsville Hospital. It was the nearest hospital to Red Plains, about 40 miles away.

Doc was married for 35 years. He and his wife had three

children, each of whom got married and moved to nearby cities or towns. Doc and his wife would visit with his grandchildren and great grandchildren every so often. His wife died ten years ago, so he now lived alone in an apartment a few blocks from his office. Doc Ford walked to work each morning.

*

Connor and Andrea Mateo both grew up in Collinsville but moved to Red Plains shortly after they got married. They knew each other in high school. Connor was four years older than Andrea; they met through Connor's younger sister. Connor had been to Red Plains many times. He used to play baseball against the Red Plains High School team. Connor went to college and got a degree in finance. Andrea was just finishing high school when they were married. Andrea was a marginal student and did not have the ambition or finances to go to college. Soon after the wedding, Connor got a job at one of the local banks in Red Plains. Andrea stayed at home. They were trying to have a baby. It didn't take long. Andrea got pregnant within four months of moving to Red Plains. She took good care of herself during the pregnancy. She neither smoked cigarettes nor drank alcohol. She went to an obstetrics clinic back in Collinsville.

Peggy-Sue Mateo was born during the summer. She was born four weeks early, and weighed just 3 pounds 4 ounces. Shortly after birth, she was jaundiced and was put into an incubator for three days where she received ultra-violet light therapy, a common treatment for premature infants. This reduced the yellow pigment in her skin due to bilirubin, a hemoglobin breakdown product. She also developed fetal respiratory distress syndrome due to an insufficient production of surfactants in her lungs. These detergent-like chemicals increase the surface area of the lungs and help keep the integrity of newborn lungs. Both of the conditions that Peggy-Sue had were the result of her prematurity. For the first 14 days of her life, she was hospitalized with respiratory problems. Her body weight was in the lowest 25th percentile at two weeks, when she was discharged from the hospital and sent home.

Three weeks after her birth, Peggy-Sue developed dehydration, fever, and an overall failure to thrive. Her parents drove her to the Collinsville Hospital. Dr. Ford happened to be the physician on duty that afternoon. He examined Peggy-Sue and determined that she had a cold. He prescribed 1 cc of Bromatane, to be taken every four hours. She spent the next few days in the hospital, where she gradually improved and was discharged. Dr. Ford told Andrea to keep giving Bromatane to her daughter after discharge.

Seven days later, Peggy-Sue became lethargic and unresponsive; a red liquid was coming from her nose. Andrea called emergency medical services, who tried to revive the child. Unfortunately, she had already passed. Peggy-Sue's small body was taken from the family, wrapped in her blanket, and sent to the morgue. Connor did his best to console his grieving wife.

Because the death occurred unexpectedly, an autopsy was ordered. It was performed by pathologists hired by the county coroner's office. There were no physical abnormalities with the body itself, only that she was small for her age. Toxicology tests were ordered. When the results came back a few days later, they revealed the presence of pseudoephedrine and brompheniramine, consistent with the Bromatane medication that was prescribed to her. But the concentrations were in the toxic range at 755 and 68 ng/mL, respectively. The pathologist ruled that the drugs from these cold medications likely contributed to her death.

The funeral was held three days later in Red Plains. Most of the town came out to pay their last respects to the infant, including Doc Ford and his staff at the office. Nobody seemed to blame Doc Ford for the death of Peggy-Sue. This was a tight community that knew how to protect their own residents. Doc Ford was considered a member of everyone's family in Red Plains. He brought many lives into the world here, and saved many others.

Since Connor Mateo did not grow up in Red Plains, he did not have the same attitude toward the town's doctor. He contacted Dennis McCaffrey, an attorney from Collinsville regarding negligence in the death of his daughter. When word got out that Connor was having someone investigate Doc Ford's medical practices, people started saying bad things about Connor behind his back. His co-workers at the bank started giving him the cold shoulder. "How could he think that Doc Ford caused this?" one of them said to another.

"Was the dosage given to my daughter typical?" Connor asked Mr. McCaffrey in his law office.

"That is what we will have to find out. I'll contact pediatricians from outside Red Plains to be sure. I also know a toxicologist from the General Hospital who may be able to give us an opinion as to the drug levels found in Peggy-Sue's blood," McCaffrey said.

I got the call from McCaffrey and agreed to take the case. Having three children of my own, these cases were particularly troubling to me. There have been other cases of doctors indiscriminately using over-the-counter cold medications in a pediatric population, thinking that they were safe.

"Infants and children are particularly difficult to manage therapeutically," McCaffrey's pediatrician expert told McCaffrey and me. "Medications designed for adults and older children have to be used with extreme caution. Sometimes it is best to just hydrate and not medicate, and to let a cold take its course. But it is a delicate balance," he concluded.

As someone involved with pharmacology, I added to the discussion. "While it's true that toddlers and young children have a higher metabolic rate than adults, which necessitates higher dosages per unit of body weight, it's just the opposite with premature infants. Because their liver enzymes are not fully developed, they need substantially less medication than toddlers. In the case of Peggy-Sue, she was four weeks premature and died at four weeks of life. Therefore she was basically a newborn, not a one-month old infant."

The post mortem toxicology data was sent to me for my evaluation. From the literature, I told McCaffrey that the pseudoephedrine concentration was within the range of 700 to 13,000 that was reported for other deaths. For brompheniramine, the result was within the lower range of 50-900 of previously reported deaths.

"I think we have enough to take this to trial," I said.

To McCaffrey, this case appeared to be fairly straightforward. The Physicians' Desk Reference, an authoritative text on medications, stated: "Do not use this in newborns, premature infants, and in nursing mothers." So it came as a big surprise to McCaffrey that the defendant's lawyer, Jerry Singleton, rejected the settlement offer and instead opted for a jury trial.

"Jerry has something up his sleeve," McCaffrey told me. There were only a few law offices in the vicinity of Red Plains, so every lawyer knew and opposed each other many times.

The defense hired their own pharmacology expert witness to refute the conclusions rendered by the medical examiners. Dr. Hannah Steffen was an adjunct clinical professor of pharmacology. During a pretrial deposition, she said, "Given the half-life of the two drugs, pseudoephedrine and brompheniramine, the amount of drug found at the time of the child's death could not have been the result of the prescribed dosage. We therefore conclude that Mrs. Mateo must have given her child additional drug doses that led to Peggy-Sue's death."

"Dr. Steffen, Andrea Mateo vehemently denies giving her child medications not prescribed by Dr. Ford. We have the original bottle containing Peggy Sue's prescription and can prove that there are no dosages missing," McCaffrey countered.

"That doesn't exclude the possibility of her getting drugs from other sources" Dr. Steffen said.

"Red Plains is a small town," said McCaffrey. "We checked all the pharmacies in the area to see if there was any record of Bromatane purchases by the Mateo family. Under a witness by the Red Plains police, we also searched the family home for other bottles of Bromatane. They found none."

Dr. Steffen responded, "We're not suggesting that the family gave the child more Bromatane, but rather that she was given a medication that only contained pseudoephedrine. The postmortem blood level for pseudoephedrine was disproportionately higher than brompheniramine. Moreover, the forensic lab reported no dextromethorphan. If this was an overdose of the Bromatane that she was prescribed, where is the third drug?"

After the deposition, McCaffrey called me in to discuss this new development. He told me, "We cannot go to trial because we will lose this case. How can we counter these arguments?"

I responded, "I have to see the laboratory's original data to see if there is any evidence of dextromethorphan in Peggy-Sue's postmortem blood. It may be that the concentration was too low for the lab to report it."

The pathologist at the coroner's office had sent postmortem blood to a national toxicology laboratory that performed the testing. I knew the lab director, so I called him to get the instrument readouts I was seeking. The testing was conducted by gas chromatography and mass spectrometry. In reviewing the data from Peggy-Sue's file, I saw that there was an extra blip or peak that could have been due to the missing drug. I asked the lab to re-examine the data for the presence of dextromethorphan. The lab director called a few hours later and was embarrassed to tell me that his lab had made a mistake by overlooking this extra compound. His lab prepared and faxed an amended report to indicate that methorphan was present at 300 ng/mL. *This is the third ingredient in Bromatane. It was there all the time,* I said to myself. A level of 300 is considered toxic.

During pre-trial motions, Singleton had argued that the

case had to be moved out of the county. "We will not be able to find an impartial jury in this small town," he argued. McCaffrey agreed and the case was moved to Fresno, California. The trial began and the plaintiff presented their case first.

I was put on the stand to testify regarding the toxicologic analysis. "From the amended toxicology report, it is now evident that dextromethorphan was present at toxic levels in Peggy-Sue's blood at the time of her death. We opine that the typical half-life of medications given to adults is increased dramatically when it comes to infants, particularly premature babies. In other words, the rate of drug breakdown and removal from the body is greatly reduced, resulting in toxic accumulation. We have several lines of independent evidence that Peggy-Sue was premature at the time of her birth.

"What is this evidence?" McCaffrey asked, knowing full well the answer to his question.

I proceeded. "First, she was born four weeks early and had a low birth weight. Second, she had high serum bilirubin concentrations that required treatment with ultra-violet light. A mature liver is needed to process bilirubin. Third, she was born with respiratory distress syndrome. She did not have the surfactants needed to breathe on her own when she was born," I concluded.

McCaffrey then asked, "Mrs. Mateo has testified that she did not give her child any additional medication. The investigators found no other sources of drugs. Andrea Mateo is an inexperienced, first-time mother. She would not go against the medical advice of her doctors. Assuming this information is accurate, do you, doctor, have an opinion as to the cause of death?"

"She died of an overdose of Bromatane," I concluded.

The defense attorney asked the judge for a recess and a meeting to discuss terms with McCaffrey and the Mateo family. The defense's assertion that an additional drug was given to Peggy-Sue by her mother was proven false. McCaffrey asked for a generous settlement award. Jerry Singleton convinced Dr. Ford to accept the offer.

"We have one further stipulation," McCaffrey said to Singleton. "Dr. Rupert Ford must retire from his medical practice. At age 84, he is no longer able to protect the interests of the community," McCaffrey stated. All Jerry Singleton could do at this stage was to nod his head. He didn't want Doc to treat his child after trying this case.

Dr. Ford realized that his actions caused the death of this poor child. He told his staff, Betty and Priscilla, that he must retire.

"It's time for me to let the next generation take over," he said. Actually, it was time for the generation after the next generation to take over. The defense accepted the terms, and Dr. Ford vacated his practice. Six months later, the town held a celebration of Doc Ford's life and career. Thousands of people he had treated came back to Red Plains for the festivities. It was a gala that only a small town can appreciate. A new doctor came to town two years later to take over Doc Ford's practice. Doc died within a year after his retirement. This sometimes happens to people who dedicate themselves to a singular goal. For example, Joe Paterno, the Penn State University football coach for over 50 years died shortly after *his* dismissal. Connor transferred to a job at the bank branch in Collinsville. He and Andrea moved there and had another baby two years later.

*

The assumption that an over-the-counter medication is safe is not correct. This is particularly true when the recommendations on the package inserts are ignored. There has been an increasing incidence of deaths due to cold medications. The dosage of the active ingredients for some of these medications has increased in recent years. Labeling such as "extra strength" and "fast relief" are making these drugs more dangerous to the unsuspecting consumer, as they usually contain a higher drug concentration than "regular strength." In our fast-paced society the need and desire to "get well fast" has its price.

Premature infants are a particularly vulnerable population because of the slow maturation of their liver enzymes. There are currently no laboratory tests to access metabolic rates. Gestational and chronologic ages are the only indicators of prematurity, and they are crude at best. Due to significant advances in neonatal medical care, higher numbers of infants are born prematurely. They are surviving with shorter and shorter in utero gestation duration. Medical and therapeutic strategies designed for full-term infants are not applicable to premature babies.

Intentional abuse of over-the-counter medication has become a problem for teenagers and young adults. Drugs such as dextromethorphan are readily available and can produce a hallucinogenic high. Street names include Robo, Dex, Tussin, Skittles, and Red Hots. In the U.S, 41 states have enacted legislation that makes it more difficult to purchase pseudoephedrine from pharmacies. In addition to requiring proper identification and the tracking of purchases, there are limits as to the amount that can be bought at any given time. Currently, clinical laboratories do not have assays for testing for the abuse of cold medications. Therefore, abuse must be suspected by clinical presentation, and urine samples tested by reference toxicology laboratories.

I was saddened to have participated in the forced retirement and eventual death of a physician who had dedicated his life to medical practice. It is very difficult to get new doctors to live and work in small towns, hence there is a shortage. Nevertheless, Doc was no longer competent and a change in the community was needed.

No Snack for Yew

****

Lincoln "Skip" Hastings III was a highly ambitious man from a highly competitive family. It began with his grandfather, Lincoln Hastings I, and his father, Lincoln Hastings II. In 1978, after President Jimmy Carter legalized the private brewing of beer in one's own home, Skip's father and grandfather formed Hastings Brewery, one of the first microbreweries in the U.S. Skip was a teenager at the time. Within five years, Skip's grandfather retired, and 10 years later, so did his father, so at age 33, Skip became CEO of the brewery.

Skip was married to Clara and had two sons, Lincoln Hastings IV, or "Link," and Darrell. They lived in a large house on the outskirts of the city. Like his father before him, Skip did not spend a lot of time with his sons. He did, however, plan that they would enter the business after he retired.

When Clara was in her late thirties, she unexpectedly became pregnant with their third child. Link and Darrell were 14 and 12 at the time. Because of Clara's age, her obstetrician, Dr. Holly Wallace, recommended that she undergo prenatal testing for birth defects so that decisions as to whether or not to continue the pregnancy could be made. Initially, her blood was collected during her second trimester and tested for the "triple markers" — alpha fetoprotein, unconjugated estriol, and human choriogonodotropin, or hCG. These tests examine a woman's likelihood of carrying a baby with Down syndrome, neural tube defects such as spina bifida, and other abnormal newborn conditions. If the unborn child has any genetic deficiencies, these can be uncovered with this testing and decisions regarding whether to continue the pregnancy or not can be made. Clara's result suggested a high likelihood for Down syndrome. As a next step, her doctor recommended amniocentesis for chromosomal analysis. A long needle was poked into her stomach and a small amount of fluid from the gestational sac was removed. The chromosomal analysis revealed an X and a Y chromosome, meaning that she was carrying another boy. Unfortunately, the fetus also had "trisomy 21," three separate copies of the number 21 chromosome.

"What does that mean for us?" Clara asked Dr. Wallace. Skip was out of town on a business meeting and not present for this discussion.

"It means that your child will develop Down syndrome," Dr. Wallace replied. "It is likely that he will have some degree of mental disability and will be dependent for much of his life."

"Is there any cure?" Clara wasn't sure if she wanted to raise a child who would be developmentally challenged, and she wanted more information to be able to make an informed decision. Clara and Skip were having marital problems before this pregnancy. But Skip promised his mother before she died that he would keep his family intact.

"No, there isn't a cure," said Dr. Wallace. "But I can tell you that many children with Down syndrome lead productive lives."

Clara thanked the doctor for taking the time to answer all of her questions, and left the office. She called Skip with the news. When she explained to him that their son may be mentally challenged, Skip delicately asked Clara if she would be willing to have an abortion.

"Absolutely not," she said. "We have the financial means to raise and care for this child. You will not take this baby from me." She was hoping that a new child would bring them closer together again like they'd been when their other sons were young. But the prospect of caring for a Down syndrome child irrevocably fractured their marriage.

The remainder of Clara's pregnancy was unremarkable, Skip was never again intimate with Clara. She moved down the hallway into her own bedroom at the house. Skip threw himself more and more into his work, and began taking his sons to work with him. Clara delivered a baby boy with Down syndrome. He was named Willow.

In the meantime, Skip began seeing Brea, his executive secretary. There was no secret to his infidelity. Brea was young and pretty, and made it clear to Skip that she wanted him. Brea lived in a downtown apartment financed by Skip, where he was a frequent guest. After a few years, Brea begged him to divorce Clara, but Skip refused.

Willow was a happy and loving child, although he was slow to develop physically and mentally. He didn't start walking until he was two, and didn't speak cogently until he was three. Clara tried, with no success, to engage him with other children his age. He was not inquisitive about his surroundings. He largely accepted the care that was offered to him. But he appeared to be happy. He didn't cry a lot and never complained. His older brothers would play with him, but as they got older they got busier with their activities and had increasingly less time for him.

Clara's love for Willow was very different than for her other sons. His presence filled a void left by her failed marriage and then by her sons' departures for college. Clara liked the fact that Willow was dependent on her. As fate would have it, however, Clara developed a lump in her breast and was diagnosed with breast cancer. Because she was so consumed with Willow, she'd put off her annual mammography screening, and her diagnosis came too late. She was treated with a lumpectomy and chemotherapy, but her tumor metastasized to her liver. Just before she passed away, she begged Skip for one last favor.

"Please don't move Willow to a home, "she said. "He is happy here. This is his home. He has never lived anywhere else. He has known no other life and it will be difficult for him to cope if he isn't here." Skip promised her that he would not force Willow to leave.

Skip was genuinely saddened by Clara's death. Although he knew she was dying, when it actually happened, he took it harder than he thought he would. He loved her during the first years of their marriage. Her death opened the door for Brea. Skip hired a woman to live in the house and care for Willow in their home. Skip and Brea waited for a period of mourning and then got married within six months after Clara's passing. Brea didn't take the time to know or love Willow. She was hoping for her own family with Skip. She pleaded with him to move Willow to a home with other children with Down syndrome.

"Willow isn't happy here by himself," she said. "He needs to be with other children that are like him. They have programs that can cater to his special needs." None of this was true; she just wanted to have him out of their lives. Skip did not want to break his promise to his first wife. But Brea said, "Let's at least take a look at the place that I've found."

So they scheduled a visit to the Evergreen Home, a facility specializing in children with Down syndrome and autism. Skip investigated the home on the Internet and found that it was very highly rated. Written comments on Yelp included "Very clean." "Landscape immaculately manicured." "Lots of open spaces for children to run around." And most important, "Residents are lovingly cared for." Skip made an appointment and met with Ms. Phyllis Hamilton, the headmistress. The family ate lunch together at the home and the food was excellent. In the cafeteria, there were kids there of all ages, all of whom appeared to be happy. Before Brea and Skip sat down with Phyllis, the headmistress bent down and asked Willow, "Honey, do you want to go out and play with the other children while we adults talk?"

Willow was shy at first and hung onto Skip's leg. But when he saw the other kids yelling and shouting while they were outside playing a game of tag, he decided to join them. After Willow left, Phyllis talked about life at Evergreen.

"We keep careful watch over our residents. There is an onsite nurse and a doctor on call 24 hours a day with regular health exams for everyone. We have an active physical education program. Some of our residents have participated in the local Special Olympic Games. Our educational program has won awards for its progressive approach in teaching vocational skills. We have an excellent record of job placement for residents once they have reached adulthood. Some have even gotten married."

Skip was very pleased with what he saw at the Evergreen Home. But he didn't want to make a hasty decision. Phyllis did not pressure Skip to make one, either.

Instead she said, "You are welcome to bring Willow back at any time to get to know the other kids. If you like, we can even arrange for a sleepover. Everything will be supervised as it always is."

So Skip brought Willow back three more times over the course of the next few months. Each time, he and Willow would stay a little longer. On the third visit, Willow stayed over a Saturday night. When Skip came back Sunday morning to pick up Willow, Skip saw that the visit had gone well. Willow was busy playing games with some of the other kids.

"Oh, hi Dad. This is Peppy, my friend." Willow didn't seem to be in a hurry to go home. Skip could see that Willow was getting along nicely with the other kids and coming out of his shell. Over the course of the last few weeks of visiting the home, Willow was growing emotionally. When they returned home, Skip asked Willow if he wanted to live at the Evergreen Home full time with the other children. Skip asked Brea not to be present for this talk.

"Will you come and visit me, Dad?" Willow asked.

"Of course. And Grandad, Link, and Darrell would come to see you too," Skip said.

"Okay, Dad. I like it there. There is one kid who is younger than me who follows me around all the time. We've become friends."

"You're sure, Willow?" Skip asked.

"Yeah, I'm sure. What's for lunch?" Willow asked.

Skip signed the papers and Willow Hastings, age nine, moved into Evergreen the following week.

Skip tried to keep his promise to his son as much as possible. He visited Willow as often as his work allowed. But it was clear that Evergreen was caring for Willow's every need and that Skip's visits, though welcomed, were not really necessary. In the meantime, Brea became pregnant and gave birth to twin baby girls. Skip was starting his third round of children.

Willow lived at Evergreen Home for several years without any incident. Then one day, inexplicably, he started eating leaves and flowers from the garden. Willow was slightly obese as many Down syndrome children are, so his behavior wasn't out of malnutrition or hunger. He liked salads and thought that the decorative plants were edible, as well. None of the staff saw Willow chewing on these plant materials, so nobody stopped him.

At first there were no medical consequences. But one day, he developed severe stomach cramps followed by a seizure in the lounge. Caretakers saw this and immediately called the doctor who told them to take Willow to the hospital immediately. Evergreen Home also called Skip who said that he would meet them at the hospital. In the emergency department, an electrocardiogram showed that Willow had ventricular tachycardia; his heart was beating at a rapid rate. Shortly thereafter, his heart stopped. He was immediately given epinephrine, succinylcholine, lidocaine, and calcium. The doctors attempted to defibrillate with 200, then 300 and finally 360 joules but to no avail. Willow died before his father and stepmother arrived at the hospital.

Willow's body was sent to the morgue where an autopsy was performed. In his lungs, they found a blood clot in the proximal portions of a pulmonary artery. In his leg, there was another clot that lodged just above his Achilles tendon. The medical examiner concluded that Willow died of a pulmonary embolus that broke free from a blood clot in a leg vein and lodged upstream into the pulmonary artery.

Skip read the autopsy report. He was stopped by the finding about Willow's stomach at the time of death. It read, "The stomach contains about 300 milliliters of a greenish/tan fluid with fragments of fine conifer-like needles and dark green plant/vegetable matter. There are also some red berry-like materials. The cecal region contains softer tan fecal material containing fine flat green flecks of plant-like material." Skip also read that a friend had seen Willow eating plants in the garden just before his death.

Could eating these plants have caused his blood clot?" Skip wondered. He put in a call to Duane McVey, a former police detective who was a private investigator.

"I want to know what happened at the Home on the day my son died," Skip told him. I'm not suspecting any foul play, but I promised his mother that I would look out for him before she died, and I feel like I let her down."

Once on the case, McVey requisitioned the emergency medical technician's report, records from the hospital, and autopsy report from the medical examiner. When he read about

Willow eating plants, he went to the Evergreen Home and talked with Phyllis Hamilton. Skip particularly wanted McVey to find out about the plant Willow had been eating. McVey and the headmistress questioned some of Willow's friends and found one who had seen him outside the day he died. The boy took them out in the courtyard and showed them what plant Willow had consumed. McVey took a picture of the shrub, snipped off a part of the plant needles, and removed some of the red berries before leaving the Home.

McVey called Skip. "I have some of the shrub your son was eating at the time of his passing. The gardener says it is Japanese Yew. I've contacted a toxicologist at the General Hospital, who is working on the case."

"Proceed with your investigation," Skip told him.

When I got the call from McVey, I admitted that I knew little about plant poisons, but that I had a colleague at the Poison Center who did. Together, McVey and I met with Dr. Fran Mussa. "The toxic ingredient in Japanese Yew is an alkaloid called taxine," Dr. Mussa explained. "This chemical was used to produce paclitaxel, a chemotherapeutic drug. These medications are highly toxic to tumors, and as a result, to normal tissues as well. Taxines have been reported to produce respiratory depression and an abnormal slowing of the heart rate."

"But he had a rapid heart rate at the time of death Doc," McVey said.

"Yeah, so that doesn't really fit," said Dr. Mussa.

"So what does it all mean, Doc?" McVey asked.

"Sometimes a toxin can have a paradoxical effect. The exact opposite of what is expected." Dr. Mussa then turned to me and said, "If you can show that Willow had a high concentration of taxine A in his body, it would help us determine if it contributed to his death."

With that assignment, I contacted the medical examiner's office to see if there were any remaining tissues or body fluids from the autopsy of Willow Hastings. The pathologist assistant told me that there was no urine or liver tissue taken, and there were only a few drops of blood left. We tried to determine if taxine was present, but in the end, there just weren't enough samples left.

I sent a report to Duane McVey, who conveyed this information to Willow's father. In my report, I wrote, "We cannot prove that Willow's eating the yew plant had anything to do with his death. But given that the Evergreen Home serves mentally challenged patients, it is inappropriate to have these plants on their grounds. Pica, or chewing on inedible materials, is a common disorder among this population." Skip thanked both McVey and me for our investigational work.

Skip then contacted Phyllis to tell her of the conclusions and of the potential poison that was contained within the Evergreen Home's garden. "Phyllis, your Home took great care of my son and I will be forever grateful. But I suggest that you remove Japanese Yew from your property so that there is no trouble with any of the other children. My personal accountant will be writing you a check for $100,000 as a charitable donation to your Evergreen Home. I hope that you will use some of this money to alter the landscaping around the Home." Phyllis was grateful for Skip's contribution. She had the Home's landscaper remove the yew plants and replace them with palms and a

fountain. The area was named "Willow's Tranquility Garden."
Skip, Brea, and the twins were hosts for the grand opening.

*

*Besides certain mushrooms, there are several other plants that are
poisonous to humans. According to the 2009 Annual Report of the
American Association of Poison Control Centers' National Poison Data
System, the top three most frequently reported plant species causing
toxicity in humans were 1) Spathiphylum, such as the Peace Lily; 2)
Phytolacca Americana, including pokeweed and American nightshade;
and 3) Toxicodendrons, including poison ivy, oak, and sumac. Others
include cardiac glycoside-containing plants, colchicum autumnalis, ricin,
and abrin.*

*Yew plants are also toxic, although very few deaths attributed
to this have ever been reported to the Poison Control Centers. While the
toxin contained in yew plants appears to be more dangerous to chickens,
dogs, and cows than to humans, both the needles and berry seeds of the
plant are toxic and can produce gastrointestinal pain and convulsions as
seen in Willow's case.*

*Pica is a relative common psychiatric disorder characterized by
having an appetite for non-nutritional substances, which can lead to
serious   medical   consequences.   Children   with   developmental
abnormalities have the highest incidence of pica. For example, a number
of children have developed lead poisoning by eating paint chips or flakes.
While lead in house paint was banned in 1978 by the U.S. Consumer
Product Safety Commission, there are still many old buildings and
apartments whose walls are covered with lead paint.*

*Because the incidence of birth defects increases dramatically
with advancing age, the triple marker test is widely used as a screening*

75

test for women who will be over 35 at the time of delivery. In 2007, the American College of Obstetrics and Gynecology recommended that all women need to be offered, at a minimum, the option to undergo triple marker testing. This gives women more options in terms of pregnancy termination or planning for the care of the child. Some clinical laboratories have added a fourth serum test, inhibin A, to improve the predictive value of the triple marker test, particularly for Down syndrome and trisomy 18. These children typically experience developmental delays and may have structural birth defects to their heart, kidneys, and gastrointestinal tract.

Dumbing It Down

****

Rusty Witt was always the smartest kid in school. Most of it came very naturally to him. His father attributed his genius to his photographic memory. He could read a page of text by visualizing it, scanning it in his brain and committing it to memory, much like a computer. Then he could go back through his mind and re-read the stored image with his eyes closed. Rusty's father, Mitchell, recognized that his son had a special gift very early in the boy's life. He found out about this when they were on vacation. The family was driving in their car and looking for their hotel. Rusty was just 2 and a half years old. Rusty's mother, Regina had a brochure from the hotel and was showing it to her husband when they were at a stop light.

Rusty saw the picture while seated in the car seat between them and spoke out. "Mommy, we just passed the hotel." Rusty then proceeded to describe where it was and details of what he had seen, including the colors of the flowers adorning the entrance, the number of cars in the parking lot, and even the number of windows that the hotel had facing the street. What was more amazing was that Rusty just learned how to count a few months ago. When they arrived at the hotel, Mitchell stopped the car in front of the property. It took them 10 minutes, but he and his wife verified that what Rusty said was completely accurate.

They were dumbfounded and totally speechless for the first few moments.

Mitchell began stuttering but eventually said to his wife, "There, ah, there are no flowers in the photo you have and, and, he could not have known how many cars are in the parking lot." The father then turned to Rusty and asked, "Son, how did you, I mean, um, how did you know how many cars were in the parking lot?"

"I can see them all so I count them, Daddy" the child said.

"But we drove by the hotel quickly, dear. You didn't have time to count," Regina said.

The family car was now under the driveway away from the parking lot. "I can see them now" the boy said. "There is a blue car next to a red car, a truck, and empty space...."

From that moment on, Mitchell and Regina knew that their son was going to be very different from the other children. When he was 8 years old, they sat down with him and explained that he had a special skill in seeing and remembering things that other children and people could not do. They told him that he had to keep this a secret, because others might not understand and try to take advantage of his skill. It was ok to be smart, but they wanted him to have a normal childhood and lead a normal life. Mitchell thought that his child was sort of like Clark Kent, but Rusty was not from another planet and didn't have superhuman powers. Just a brain that had talents few others possessed.

Rusty continued to exhibit a photographic memory throughout his childhood. He took his advice and never bragged about this talent or tried to benefit from it other than through his school work. He wanted to be just another kid from the neighborhood. But his grades were so good that he was able to skip a few grades. But by the time he was 16 years, he was ready to enter college. Rusty got early acceptance to attend the State University. To celebrate his last summer before college, his parents took their only child on a family vacation to a Greek island. They booked a private tour and drove around spectacular cliffs. Rusty had seen pictures of the island views from travel books and compared the scene outside the van's window to his memory of the photos.

"The ocean is even more deep blue in reality than in the pictures" he told his mother.

Then a few minutes later, Rusty saw that there was an oncoming car and was headed straight for the van. "Watch out!" he shouted. Their van driver veered off to the left and avoided the vehicle. In doing so, however, the van slid off the road and tumbled into a ravine. The van did three rollovers before coming to a stop. The family was thrown about within the vehicle. Rusty suffered some broken bones and both he and the van driver suffered a severe concussion and were taken to a hospital. Both of his parents and their tour guide were crushed by the roof and died on the scene. Rusty was unconscious for several months while in a Greek hospital intensive care unit. His medical costs were covered by the tour's insurance policy. When he awoke from his coma, he remembered the car coming towards him, but had no recollection of the accident itself. When he was told that his parents perished in the accident, he went into a deep depression. While Rusty recovered in the Greek hospital, he was visited by his Uncle Robert, Mitchell's older brother, who became Rusty's guardian. When his health stabilized, Uncle Robert flew his nephew back to the U.S. Rusty stayed at his uncle's home for the next 12 months recovering from his injuries. The boy suffered several broken ribs and a fractured collarbone. He postponed starting college until the following fall. The school had no problem with the postponement given the extenuating circumstances. Although all of his bones healed, Rusty would get migraine headaches that required medication. Drugs seemed to help him get through each day. The car accident did not affect Rusty's memory or intelligence. In the fall of the following year, some 15 months after that tragic event, he was ready to start college. Uncle Robert gave him an old used car and told him he could come back to his home at any time. Rusty was appreciative with his Uncle's support. When Rusty finally arrived at school, he was still a year younger at 17 than most of his classmates and eager to move on with his life.

Rusty adjusted well to college life. Keeping busy helped him ease the pain of his parent's deaths. But the medication he was taking did not stop his headaches. A few months after starting school, he went back to his family physician and asked for an alternative medication to take for his migraines. He was given a prescription for a different analgesic drug, which seemed to help. Rusty wanted to lead a normal college life, so now that he was feeling better, he started to go out to college parties on weekends. Beer was present at many of these gatherings but Rusty was told that he had to avoid alcohol because of the medications he was taking. One of the parties he attended was at a fraternity that he was interested in pledging. As the evening wore on, Rusty became dizzy and confused. He wanted to say that he needed to go back to the dorm to rest, but he had difficulty verbalizing this to his friends. Instead, he just stared at them trying to formulate words. The other boys naturally thought he was drunk. When it was time to leave, they accompanied Rusty back to his room without speaking. The next day, nobody gave what happened the previous night a second thought.

Rusty didn't know it at the time, but this episode at the party was just the beginning of his cognitive decline. In class, he started losing his focus. His mood changed from one of curiosity to indifference. His mind began to wonder when his instructors were lecturing. He started thinking to himself, "*What is the matter with me? Pay attention!*" But it didn't help, many of his classes such as chemistry required synthesis of ideas instead of simple rote memorization. For the first time in his life, he got grades of "Bs" on his exams instead of "As". Rusty sought help from the guidance counselor. But when he came into the office, the counselor had seen it all before in other students and she was of no help.

"Excellence in high school doesn't always translate into the same dominance in college" she told Rusty. "The coursework is much more difficult. Your fellow classmates, especially at this school, are much smarter than your former contemporaries. You can no longer get straight As without studying. Perhaps your work habits are not as good as they need to be because you never had to study hard to succeed before."

Rusty wanted to rebut her statements but he couldn't get the words out. So he simply nodded his head and left the office.

81

Rusty was very upset and insulted at the same time. He knew he was a good student and his study habits were not the problem. There was something organically wrong with his brain. *Maybe I should seek medical help,* he thought to himself. *But who do I turn to?* This gradual cognitive decline continued for the next few weeks.

Rusty needed a break from school. He called Uncle Robert and told him he was driving home for the weekend. He took his usual drug dose in the dorm room, but forgot to put the bottle of pills it in his suitcase and headed home on a Saturday morning. After a few hours, he stopped for lunch at a small town. He pulled up to the diner but rather than parking, he made a sharp turn and began to drive onto the sidewalk. Startled pedestrians dove out of the vehicle's way to avoid getting hit. A number of people started shouting at him to stop and get off the walkway. Rusty did not hear or see them and continued driving at a slow rate. He was dazed and confused. Eventually, he ran into a traffic stoplight pole that halted his vehicle. The airbag deployed onto his head and face. Rusty was not injured. He passed out and slumped onto the empty passenger seat. None of the pedestrians were struck by the vehicle, although one elderly woman fell to the ground trying to avoid the car. An ambulance was called and both he and the fallen woman were taken to the General Hospital.

The doctor attending to Rusty was Stewart Carver, who called me to discuss the unusual case of a college student driving onto the sidewalk. The blood alcohol and usual drugs of abuse testing such as cocaine, methamphetamine, heroin, and marijuana were negative. Because the boy was unconscious. his medication history was not immediately available. There were

82

also no drugs or pills found in his car or on his clothing. Blood and urine were sent to my laboratory for a comprehensive drug screen. Our initial focus was for hallucinogens, including phencyclidine, LSD, mescaline, ketamine, even psychedelic mushrooms. None of them were present. We did, however, find the drug topiramate. This is not a drug that we normally observe among patients who are admitted to a hospital. We reported the result to Dr. Carver. I then asked one of my students, Marie Ann, to do a quick literature search on the potential side effects of the drug. The next day, we paged Dr. Carver to discuss our lab findings.

"Dr. Carver, is our topiramate patient awake yet?" I asked.

"Yes, I am in his room right now. The nurse told me that he awoke early this morning. He is confused as to what happened to him and he wants some answers."

"I'll be right there" I replied to Dr. Carver.

When I arrived at the hospital, the doctor and Uncle Robert were in the room with Rusty. Dr. Carver had already begun asking some of the questions that I wanted to ask. For example, he asked his uncle if he felt his nephew was behaving strangely. He stated that Rusty was always the best student in school and that his performance of late had declined. Rusty also asked Dr. Carver if he knew what was wrong with him. Dr. Carver said it was likely the drug he was taking.

This was a cue to me to explain further. "There have been research reports indicating that a fraction of patients taking topiramate have some decline in cognitive function and impaired verbal fluency. While the levels of topiramate in your blood appear to be within acceptable limits, you may be one of the patients prone to this side effect." Knowing that he was a good student, I gave him a copy of a research study that my staff downloaded. "How long have you been on this medication?" I asked.

Rusty replied that his doctor changed his prescription a month ago. While this may have been more effective in treating his headaches, I suggested that it was likely the cause of his current problems of memory and speech. As Rusty's injuries were very minor, he was discharged to his Uncle's care on the next day.

Dr. Carver called Rusty's primary care physician and they agreed to use yet another anti-migraine drug. Rusty was told that the effectiveness of drugs is determined on a "trial and error" basis and not from objective evidence. "We don't know in advance what drugs will work and what won't" he told the boy.

Rusty stayed at his Uncle's house for a few more days, before returning to school. Over the next few weeks, the new medication he was prescribed made a dramatic difference in his mood and outlook. Rusty was able to focus on his school work again, and no longer had any difficulty in speaking or thinking. He was back to his old self.

About a few weeks after his hospitalization, he got a letter from the motor vehicle department. Unbeknownst to him, he got a moving traffic violation for driving under the influence of narcotics. He did not recall that a police officer had issued the citation as he was still dazed and confused at the time. The ticket indicated that he violated the state's Vehicle Code 23152(b), Driving Under the Influence (DUI) due to: "Physical or mental abilities are impaired to such a degree that the individual no longer have the ability to drive with the caution characteristic of a sober person of ordinary prudence under the same or similar circumstances." Rusty was not drunk and topiramate has not been linked to DUI before. So he called me up and asked for my help in getting out of his ticket. I agreed to be a supporting expert witness because I have testified on numerous DUI cases before. The date was set and I accompanied him to the traffic judge....

*

The medical indications of topiramate are for the treatment of seizures and for migraine headaches. There have been several research studies indicating that use of this drug alone and in combination with other medications can cause cognitive impairment. The most frequent complaint is reduced verbal fluency. There are tests used by psychologists to determine an individual's sematic memory. A subject is asked to recite as many words as possible in 60 seconds from a category, e.g., farm animals. Recalling and speaking one word, e.g., goat, will stimulate other associated words e.g., cow. These word association tests are useful in the investigation of frontal and temporal lobe areas of the brain. While verbal fluency is not associated with impaired driving, topiramate can cause sedation, dizziness, nystagmus, defined as rhythmic and oscillating movements of the eyes, and ataxia, all of which can impair driving a motor vehicle. There have been many published cases in the literature of individuals who have cognitive decline to the extent that driving is impaired. The manufacturer of the medication has given warnings regarding the operation of a motor vehicle. As with other anti-epileptic drugs, there can also be an increased risk in suicide ideation. The risk for suicide thoughts are twice those of age and gender matched controls.

Topiramate-induced side effects occur more often in women

than men, on patients who are prescribed higher than normal doses, and when the drug is used in combination with other anti-seizure medications. Rusty's impairment could not have been anticipated because he didn't fit this pattern. With a simple substitution to another drug, his mental health returned to his former state. Eventually, his migraines went away and he was weaned off all medications entirely.

Packers and Stuffers

****

Carlos and Lynn never were officially hitched, but they thought of themselves as having a common-law marriage. They had similar backgrounds involving drugs and self-indulgence. Carlos' father left his wife when Carlos was two years old, so Carlos only had a vague memory of him. His mother was a crackhead who was in and out of jail. She died of an HIV infection when he was 12. Carlos was a ward of the state until the age of 15, when he ran away from his foster home to live on the streets. Even though he had no problems with schoolwork, he stopped attending school and joined a neighborhood gang. He would say to others that they were the only family he ever had. He was in and out of trouble throughout his teenage years, stealing cars, getting into fights, and bullying people. He was no stranger to the law and was arrested on numerous occasions, spending several months in juvenile detention. He was also addicted to cocaine and heroin at an early age. In order to support his habit, he broke into houses and fenced stolen property.

Lynn lived on the other side of town. Her life was reasonably normal until her mother died of lung cancer when Lynn was ten. Her father was an abusive alcoholic. He came home in a drunken rage one day when Lynn was 12, and raped Lynn in her own bedroom thinking she was his wife. Shortly thereafter, Lynn ran away from home and lived with her aunt for the next two years. Lynn hung out with the wrong crowd. She left her aunt to live with some older girls, and then she, too, dropped out of school at 15. Her older friends, who were strippers in a seedy nightclub, took her in as sort of a little sister. But they were abusing recreational drugs and eventually got Lynn hooked as well. Soon, Lynn started stripping in the same club in order to fund her drug addiction. This eventually led her to prostitution on the streets, where she acquired a number of sexually transmitted diseases from her clientele.

While Carlos and Lynn did not know each other, their lives were each headed for ruin. They were both in their late 20s and living on the streets; their life's pattern was the same. First homelessness, then crime to purchase drugs and alcohol, then substance abuse, followed by emergency department visits and hospitalization, drug rehab centers, shelters, and then back to being homeless.

Carlos and Lynn met on the street one day by accident. It was a particularly cold night. Lynn found what appeared to be a vacant spot in an alley filled with old clothing and blankets. She lay down and tried to cover herself only to find that the space was already occupied by Carlos. They fought briefly over possession, but then realized that they were both in the same boat, and maybe could benefit from keeping each other company at least for one night. At a minimum, their bodies provided heat for one another. They spoke for a few hours that night about their lives and the mistakes they made. Lynn felt more normal than she had in a long while. In the morning, Lynn woke up to find that Carlos was gone and she was alone again. He wasn't interested in any relationships, and neither was she. They didn't see each other for several months until they ran into each other again one day at a park. They were both sober and neither was high on any drugs. Oddly enough, Lynn almost felt a little excited to see him. They sat down on a bench and enjoyed a pleasant conversation. Carlos remarked that he was sick of his life but was too cowardly to commit suicide; Lynn felt the same. They both wanted to find a way out of their situation, but didn't know how to break the vicious cycle.

During one of his drug buys, Carlos asked his pusher if there was room for him in the business. He was put in touch with the main supplier, who saw that Carlos was intelligent and could possibly sell for him. So Carlos cleaned himself up in order to be presentable and started pushing cocaine and heroin to whoever had money and needed the drugs. Sometimes it was gang members, or even high school kids, but it was all the same to Carlos. He had no remorse selling to kids. He convinced Lynn to get into the business too, and soon the couple began thinking that they could rent a room and live together, which they did a few months later. While they were still addicted to cocaine, and committing crimes, they were at least off the street and they had each other. Over the ensuing years, Carlos wanted more and more for himself and Lynn. He asked his supplier if there was something more he could do.

Ely Macer and his family had been dealing drugs and prostitutes for the past few decades. Although his activities were illegal, Ely fancied himself a businessman. He dressed in fancy clothes and drove expensive cars. He did not believe in extortion. There was plenty of money to go around and he was not interested in building a crime empire.

After working for Ely for three years, Carlos said to his employer, "I'm looking to make more money. What else can I do for your organization? I'm willing to do anything. Anything."

Ely paused and looked Carlos in the eye for several seconds trying to gauge his seriousness. When Carlos didn't blink, Ely knew he meant business. "If you want more, I can use you as a mule."

"What do I have to do?" Carlos asked.

"I need someone to transport large quantities of drugs from place to place," Ely told him. "If you get caught, you'll go to jail. There will be nothing to link you to me. My entire organization and I will deny any involvement. I'll pay you well for this work, but if you steal from me, even one ounce, you'll wish you were never born."

Carlos agreed and was given the new responsibility. At first, he was part of a group of drivers bringing drugs across state borders. He drove carefully so as to not get stopped by state troopers who could search his truck for contraband. He was careful not to be on any drugs while driving. It was important to him to keep this job, as he had no other future. If he made more money, he and Lynn could have a better life. He was paid handsomely for this work. It was easy money. Lynn knew that Carlos was likely doing something illegal. But she never asked him about it. She was just happy to be off the street.

Delivering drugs via motor vehicles was the prelude to more serious deliveries. After a year, Ely felt he could trust Carlos for the next, more important job. He told Carlos, "I want you to help us transport drugs from abroad. We will train you to be a human mule. You need to learn how to swallow pellets of cocaine and heroin. It is difficult at first and your inclination will be to gag and puke. But with practice, you'll get better at it."

"But won't swallowing large amounts of drugs be dangerous to me?" Carlos asked.

Ely said, "You have nothing to worry about. These will be professionally packaged. I guarantee they will never leak inside your body. Besides, a dead mule is of no use to me. Once you arrive back in America, these pellets will naturally pass from your body and into your poop, where we will retrieve them. I'll pay you $5,000 per trip. Do you want the job?"

Carlos was excited at the prospect of earning more money. "I'm in," he said. "Where am I going and when do I leave?"

Ely arranged for Carlos to travel to South America. He got a clean shave and a short haircut. He was given a business suit and designer shoes. He carried an expensive briefcase containing meaningless papers. He was also taught how to behave like a professional businessman. He was given a fake passport and a fictitious traveling name. These measures were all taken to draw suspicion away from the true purpose of his trip.

When Carlos arrived at his destination, Ely's contact met him at the airport with a car to take him to a hotel. Carlos knew his contact only as "Sanchez." Sanchez returned the next day carrying a package containing 72 pellets, each carefully packed to contain 10 grams of pure cocaine. Carlos prepared himself to swallow the pellets. Before proceeding, Carlos was given a warning.

"Don't mess with these guys. If you try to steal this,"

Sanchez held up the pellets to show Carlos, "they will find you anywhere in the world. This is serious business. Do what they say and you will live a long life."

Carlos was not afraid. He'd been threatened as a kid all the time. He also didn't to want to mess up a good thing. So he swallowed each pellet one by one, in full view of Sanchez. The pellets were coated with oil, making them easy to swallow. To make room in his stomach, he was instructed not to eat the night before. Only when he arrived back in the U.S. could he eat. He was told that having the pellets in his stomach would curb his appetite.

Ely was right, Carlos said to himself. *These pellets are tightly packed. There is no way these will break open.*

Sanchez and Carlos left for the airport. Carlos calmly passed through customs. The officers scanned his passport, saw nothing out of order, and let him pass. He went through the "Nothing to Declare" aisle, and within a few minutes, he was in the airport's International arrival hall. One of Ely's men was there to greet him. They took him to a hotel, where he was given a laxative. He then began to expel the pellets he had consumed. Then he was paid in cash, and went home. Lynn was happy to see him. She wasn't completely sure he would come back.

Carlos pulled out a wad of cash and said, "Let's go celebrate." Lynn didn't question where the money came from. The two of them went out to a fancy restaurant and enjoyed the best dinner they ever had.

Over the next few years, there were many more jobs for Carlos to transfer drugs from abroad. Each time, he carried a little more, and was paid a little more. He made his own travel arrangements and no longer needed anyone to meet him at the airport. He and Lynn became comfortable with their new lifestyle. They upgraded their apartment.

On his next trip to South America, Carlos was to return with his "cargo" to California. Boston was still his port of entry into the U.S. since he was familiar with customs there. Or so he thought. Lynn had never been out of the country before, and neither Lynn nor Carlos had been to the West Coast. So Carlos asked Lynn if she wanted to come. Lynn jumped at the idea. They applied for a passport in her real name.

Carlos and Lynn flew to his usual stop in South America. Carlos brought a small amount of cocaine for their personal use while they were abroad. He'd never brought any cocaine for personal use on these business trips before. They hid the drug in a cosmetics case that contained a false bottom. The couple enjoyed sightseeing and other tourist activities during the day, and got drunk on alcohol and high on cocaine at night.

On the day they were to leave, Carlos stopped drinking and snorting so that his mind would be clear when he met with Sanchez. Carlos told Lynn that it was necessary that he meet with his business associate for a few hours to discuss some matters before catching their plane back to the U.S. Lynn knew that this trip was for business, but didn't know what that business was and had been told not to ask. She wasn't particularly suspicious when Carlos said he wasn't hungry during the entire 12-hour flight home; he'd fasted for this duration before. When they arrived in Boston, Carlos saw something he had never seen before at Logan Airport. On this day, the immigration department had German Shepherds as sniff dogs circulating throughout the baggage claim area. Carlos and Lynn still carried quite a bit of cocaine hidden in the cosmetics bag remaining from their trip. According to Massachusetts law, an individual in possession of greater than 28 grams of cocaine could be convicted by the state's drug trafficking laws, with a minimum of seven years in prison. Carlos knew that they were holding more than that amount. So he took Lynn aside and told her that they had to do something about the stash.

"Let's flush it down the toilet," she said to Carlos.

"No way, this is worth a lot of money. I have a plan. We'll put it into a condom, wrap it tightly and you swallow it.

"Are you nuts? I can't do that," Lynn said.

"Don't worry; I do it all the time. In fact, I have much more than that in my stomach right now."

An astonished look came over Lynn's face. She didn't know what he did for a living, but she didn't think it was drug smuggling. Carlos then explained to Lynn how he was earning the money and how easy it was to transport cocaine. He would do it himself, he told her, but his stomach was already full. Against her better judgment, Lynn agreed. They tightly wrapped their cocaine into a new condom, and she swallowed it. The plan worked. None of the dogs at the airport could sniff the cocaine she was carrying, and they both passed through customs with no problems. Carlos and Lynn went straight to their connecting gate without exiting the airport. This way, they didn't have to pass through U.S. airport security.

The five-hour flight to California presented major problems for Lynn because a small hole developed in the condom, and cocaine began leaking into her gastrointestinal system. She started to exhibit signs of cocaine poisoning, including increased heart rate, sweating, abdominal spasms, and crushing pain to her chest. They did not disclose her symptoms to the flight attendants because they didn't want them to discover what they had done. As soon as they landed, however, they hailed a cab and told the driver to go to the nearest emergency department, which was at the General Hospital.

The triaging nurse asked them a series of questions, including recent cocaine use. Lab tests and electrocardiograms revealed that Lynn suffered a heart attack. Cocaine use was suspected because young women with no history of cardiovascular disease do not typically develop myocardial infarctions. Against Carlos' advice, Lynn admitted that she swallowed a substantial amount of cocaine to evade detection.

"I'm not going to risk my life for this," she told Carlos. She revealed that the source of her cocaine was in her stomach. A positive urine toxicology screen confirmed the presence of cocaine. The emergency room team immediately administered activated charcoal down Lynn's throat in the hope of binding any free cocaine that hadn't been ingested. She was admitted to the coronary care unit, where she recovered from her heart attack. In the meantime, Carlos went to the bathroom and excreted the pellets he had swallowed. None of them were ruptured.

But other complications soon arose. Lynn suddenly developed a dangerously low white blood cell count. Her face started breaking out with blister-like lesions. Dr. Monica Curtis, a rheumatologist, Dr. Karen Lake, a toxicologist, and I were consulted as to why this low white blood cell count might have occurred in connection with cocaine use. We went to the coronary care unit and presented our opinions to the team, which consisted of medical students, interns, residents, and other attending physicians.

"This patient has agranulocytosis with an absolute neutrophil count of less than 500 per microliters," Dr. Curtis explained. "She is at great risk for infections due to the absence of these infection-fighting cells. We need to isolate her immediately from any sources of bacteria, particularly hospital-acquired infections."

"How was this brought on by her cocaine use?" asked one of the residents.

Dr. Lake fielded to this question. "We determined that the cocaine used by this patient was cut with levamisole, a deworming agent used for large domestic animals. Illicit cocaine makers have begun adding this drug to cocaine for several years now. Up to 90% of the cocaine found on our streets has this adulterant," she explained. "Levamisole increases the heart rate, thereby improving the euphoric effects of cocaine. That's why it's added."

"If it's so prevalent, why haven't we seen more cases of agranulocytosis?" another resident asked.

"Only a small percentage of the general population is susceptible to the adverse effects of levamisole." I explained to the group. "It appears to be related to the specific types of T-cells that circulate in our blood. In other words, there is a genetic predisposition toward levamisole toxicity."

"The facial lesions may be the result of her body rejecting this chemical and is the result of an auto-immune reaction" Dr. Lake said.

While Lynn survived her heart attack, she died a few

days later of infectious complications brought on by the levamisole, despite isolation, prophylactic antibiotics, and supportive care. Having been on an airplane for more than 6 hours prior to arriving at the hospital may have added to her exposure to infectious microorganisms from fellow passengers. No charges were brought against Carlos because Lynn willingly agreed to swallow the drug. Carlos did not suffer from agranulocytosis despite the fact that he had used cocaine from the same batch as Lynn. But he did lose the only person that he'd ever cared for in his entire life.

*

One of my medical students doing a rotation at the time that Lynn was in the hospital asked me the difference between a body packer and a body stuffer and how he could remember the distinction.

I explained that a body packer is an individual who purposely smuggles drugs by oral ingestion. Like when someone is about to go on a trip, the bags are carefully packed so they are not damaged during transportation. Most body packers suffer no ill effects of the drugs they are carrying. However, if there is any breach of the bag seals, the potential for significant morbidity and mortality is high due to the large quantity of drug that is swallowed. A body packer with multiple ingested packages can often be detected by radiographic means. Airport security may have capabilities for identifying these mules.

A body stuffer, on the other hand, is an individual who ingest drugs at the last minute in order to escape detection by law enforcement. The quantity of drugs ingested is lower than what a body packer swallows. However, these packages may not be properly prepared and drug toxicities are more likely to occur. Stuffers swallowed drugs that are contained within condoms and rubber gloves.

Heart attacks induced by cocaine and methamphetamine occur through a different mechanism than those that occur naturally. In a patient with atherosclerosis, a rupture of plaque lodged onto the coronary artery stimulates a blood clot. If the artery is already narrowed by the presence of plaques, the blood clot can cause a complete blockage of the artery. A resulting cessation of blood flow causes the cardiac damage due to the lack of oxygen delivery to the heart itself. Cocaine-induced attacks are caused by the drug's ability to vasoconstrict, or narrow blood vessels. A sudden narrowing of a coronary artery can close the blood vessel thereby precipitate a heart attack even if there is not a significant degree of atherosclerosis.

Early Wakeup Call

****

Lester Popkin had it all. He was very attractive, smart, and athletic. He had his pick of the prettiest girls in school, but that didn't distract him away from his goals. From early on, he knew what he wanted and worked hard to get there. In college, he was given a full four-year basketball scholarship. As a freshman, he was the starting point guard for his college, an NCAA Division I-AA school. He made the All-Conference Team during his sophomore and junior years, and led his team to the conference title game both years. He was hoping for a chance to play professional basketball, either in Europe, the National Basketball Association's Development-League, or the NBA itself. He knew it was a long shot, but he was tall for a point guard at 6 feet 5 inches, was fast on his feet, had good hands for steals, and had a killer jump shot from behind the 3-point line. The fact that his free throw percentage hovered around 93 percent didn't hurt him either.

But the fifth game of the season of his senior year in college changed everything. It was an away game and they were playing the last of the school's non-conference schedule, a new team that he hadn't faced before. Moving without the ball was his strength, so when he saw an opening in the lane, he cut across, hoping to get a bounce pass from his off-guard teammate.

The pass was perfect; it bounced chest high and he went in for a layup. The power forward on the other team stepped into the lane to take a charge, but his arrival was late. Lester didn't see him, and they collided. When Lester fell onto his left knee, he heard a pop. He feared the worst. He ruptured an anterior cruciate ligament, and was in intense pain. The team's trainer ran onto the court. With the assistance of a teammate, Lester was carried off the court. The fans from the opposing team gave Lester a polite round of applause. His school's cheerleaders were in shock, some of them openly weeping. His season and college basketball career were over. The four-hour bus ride back to the school was the longest trip of his life. The trainer gave him some morphine but Lester was still in pain.

Lester feared that his professional basketball career was in serious jeopardy. An injury to the ACL greatly affects an athlete's ability to move side to side. In basketball, a guard is worthless unless he can defend others who are driving with the ball toward the basket. The following week, Lester underwent reconstructive knee surgery to replace his ACL. He would be on crutches for a month and have limited mobility for the first three or four months. During his convalescence, Lester was put on a variety of pain medications, including morphine, tramadol, and fentanyl. He particularly liked fentanyl because it made him feel euphoric and dissociated from his pain. It also helped him forget the life-changing situation he was facing. His injury would put doubts into the minds of professional scouts. His coaches felt that he would not be drafted by the NBA, but that it might be possible for him to latch onto a team during open tryouts in the summer.

Not wanting to live the life of a professional basketball journeyman, Lester had a plan B for his life. He had excellent grades and planned to apply to medical school since freshman year. It was only a question as to when he would apply. Now that his pro basketball career was likely over before it even started, he devoted the remainder of his senior year applying to schools for admission immediately after college rather than waiting for his athletic career to wane. He took the medical school entry exams the previous spring and scored within the ninetieth percentile. The fact that he was a division I-AA All-American athlete also helped. Medical schools are not interested in professional bookworms who only studied all day. They prefer well-rounded individuals with varying life experiences. Medical admission committee members subscribed to the belief that achievement at the highest level in one area bodes well for predicting future success in another discipline. So Lester ended up having his choice of medical schools. He ended up attending a school within the state because his fiancée, Martha, was admitted to the same institution's nursing school. They were married after Lester's first year.

During medical school, Lester had to choose between sports medicine, surgery, and anesthesiology. While he knew a lot about sports, he didn't want to be around athletes, as it reminded him too much of his own injury and how it ruined his chances for a pro basketball career. He loved surgery, but his hands were too big to get into tight spaces. So when Lester graduated from medical school, he "matched" to an anesthesiology residency at the General Hospital. This allowed him to be part of the surgical team without having to perform operations himself.

Anesthesiologists use a variety of drugs to anesthetize patients. Fentanyl is one of the drugs that are used as a local anesthetic for patients undergoing minor surgical procedures. The specific surgical area is numbed, but the patient can remain awake. Local anesthesia results in shorter recovery times. For more serious surgeries, general anesthesia is the method of choice. Patients receiving general anesthesia are unconscious for the duration of the surgery and awaken only after the procedure has ended. The anesthesiologist must administer the correct amount of drug so patients don't awaken during the procedure. Fentanyl is a potent narcotic that is sometimes used to induce an unconscious state.

As an anesthesia resident, Dr. Lester Popkin was involved each week with elective and emergency surgeries at the General. He was responsible for prescribing the type and the dosage of anesthetic drug to be used on each patient. Once the drug was received from the pharmacy, it was placed into the custody of the anesthesia staff. Having been on fentanyl during his knee injury in college, Lester was very familiar with its effects. The more Lester was administering fentanyl, the more he began thinking how easy it would be to steal a little for himself. After two years of his residency, he and Martha were growing apart. Their schedules didn't coincide and they rarely saw each other. When they were together, they were too tired for true intimacy. He needed some happiness, and thought that fentanyl could deliver it.

The drug was prepared into syringes as an injectable intravenous solution. All he had to do was to substitute some of the drug with sterile isotonic saline. Saline is a salt solution that has the same electrolyte concentration as human plasma. It is used clinically to replace fluids in patients who are dehydrated or fluid depleted. Just before his next operation, Lester took a small vial of saline and hid it under his lab coat. He also brought in an empty vial and cap to the operating prep room. From the inpatient pharmacy, Lester obtained fentanyl syringes, each labeled with the patient's name, medical record number, drug identity and concentration, and date of surgery. He shot out a few milliliters of the drug into the empty vial, and hid the unlabeled vial in his pocket. He then aspirated an equal volume of saline back into the original syringe, thereby diluting the overall fentanyl concentration.

Mr. Augustine will never miss a drop of this, he said to himself, referring to the patient who was about to have an appendectomy.

Lester recorded into the anesthesia operation notes the exact volume of fentanyl he used on each case. Because fentanyl is a Drug Enforcement Agency-listed Schedule II controlled substance, all the syringes, whether administered during surgery or not, must be returned to the inpatient pharmacy for cataloging and proper disposal. The amount of fluid remaining in the syringes must match the notes regarding the amount used for the surgery. Replacing the fentanyl solution with an equal volume of saline hid Lester's theft.

After the operation, Lester went into the scrub room to shower and change. He then went into the residents' call room with his prize. At the very back of the room, hidden by the lockers, he grabbed an empty syringe from his locker, loaded it with the fentanyl solution he'd stolen from the patient, and injected it into a vein in his arm. He then sat down and enjoyed the dissociative effect of the drug. One of the advantages of fentanyl is the drug's very short duration of action. Within the hour, the effects of the drug wore off and he was able to return to duty or go home.

Lester repeated this deception a number of times over the ensuing months. He was addicted to the drug, even though he was fully aware of its dangers. So far, nobody was the wiser. He spent less and less time at home, more and more time in the residents' room, and increasingly kept to himself.

*

Dr. Robert Derksen was the head of the anesthesia residency program at the General Hospital. He attended many anesthesia conferences where there was discussion of narcotic addiction by residents and staff. Some of the important signs of addiction included personality changes, introversion, and increased surgical workload on a voluntary basis. We never had a problem with residents abusing fentanyl before, but nobody ever expects their program to be affected.

When Dr. Derksen first met Lester during his residency interview, he found him to be engaging and extroverted. Dr. Derksen was a big college basketball fan and remembered Lester's playing days. So he took a particular interest in Lester's candidacy. But recently, he'd noted a significant change in Lester's personality and began to worry. Dr. Derksen didn't have any evidence of drug abuse so he couldn't confront him. Besides, Lester would likely deny any abuse. So instead, he called me. We previously worked together on other matters and were close colleagues.

"If I got you a fentanyl syringe from one of our cases, would you be able to test it?" Bob asked me."

"Sure, we can do that." There is always some residual amount of solution present in the syringe. Since the fentanyl concentration is much higher than what we encounter in blood or urine, our mass spectrometers have more than enough sensitivity to detect it. "Do you suspect some diversion?" I asked.

"Not really sure yet, so I don't want to tell you any of the details," Bob said. "I'll bring you a remnant syringe after the next case."

Lester's next patient was a woman undergoing spinal fusion surgery, a procedure that joined two bones together. The surgery progressed without any complications and was over in the usual amount of time. As he'd done before, Lester took this opportunity to divert some of the fentanyl in the syringe for his own abuse later that day. As per protocol, the used and unused syringes were returned to the pharmacy. Dr. Derksen asked the head pharmacist to retain the syringes from the case for testing by the laboratory. I got the call and went to pick them up. My plan was to see if the contents of the syringe used on the patient had a lower fentanyl concentration than a syringe that was prepared in the same way but was not used. The fentanyl level should be identical since they were prepared from the same stock. Anything significantly less would indicate diversion by dilution.

The next day, I asked Bob to stop by my office. There were two chromatogram printouts on my desk. "This printout is from the unused syringe and has a peak height of 15 cm," I said. The peak height is directly proportional to the fentanyl concentration. "The peak height from the used syringe is 7.5 cm, exactly half. The used syringe has been diluted. Someone has been messing with the special sauce," I told Bob, trying to ease the tension from a very serious situation.

Bob replied, "That's bad news. Are you absolutely sure?" But Bob already knew the answer to this question. What he didn't know was what he was going to do next about Lester. The decision he made would haunt Dr. Robert Derksen for the rest of his career.

The surgical schedule showed that Lester was not on call that night for any procedures. So Dr. Derksen thought he had one day before he had to pull the plug on Lester's residency. He was hoping to discuss this with the director of all residency programs at the General before confronting Lester. What he didn't know was that Lester had traded his on-call slot with another anesthesia resident that evening. So when a kidney suddenly became available for an emergency transplant operation, Lester was paged to be the anesthesiologist on the case. This transplant operation had to be started as soon as possible, because graft survival declines with each hour after the donor has died.

Marjorie Fleisher was a 45-year old patient with end-stage kidney disease due to long-standing type 1 diabetes. She had been on insulin since age 10. Her kidneys were failing so she'd been on the transplant list for several years. When a compatible donor kidney became available, she and the transplant surgeon were called into immediate action. Dr. Lester Popkin was also paged. He sent in a request for fentanyl anesthesia to the pharmacy for Marjorie's operation, and he went to work on preparing his own personal dose. Like most addicts, he became tolerant to fentanyl. It took more and more of the drug to get the same effects. So increasingly, he was substituting more of the sterile saline for the real drug. But this time, he may have gone too far.

Marjorie was prepped for the surgery. She was excited to be getting a new kidney and not be dependent on hemodialysis, with its four-hour sessions three times a week. The transplant surgeon was Dr. Dillon Bobbitt.

On the operating table, Dr. Popkin injected the fentanyl and asked Marjorie to count backwards from 100.

"100, 99, 98, 98, ...ugh, 96....," Marjorie recited and then she was out cold.

"We're ready for the incision doctor," Lester said to the surgeon who was making his final preparation for surgery. A kidney transplant is a delicate operation with many critical steps. The procedure was going well. Halfway through, however, Marjorie became increasingly conscious.

What is going on here? she thought to herself. *Why can't I open my eyes?* Her eyelids were taped shut to avoid her eyes from drying out. *Why can't I speak?* She had a breathing tube attached to her mouth and oxygen to her nose. *Get me out of here.* But she couldn't move. She was strapped to the gurney. *Help! Somebody!* After a few seconds, Marjorie's mind cleared up. *I'm on the operating table. I'm having a kidney transplant. Hooray. But I don't think I should be awake for this.* There was a pain in her lower abdomen where the incision was made to remove her damaged kidneys. *I've got to get somebody's attention.* So she started to thrash about and made some noises with her vocal chords.

The nurse noticed. "Doctors, I think the patient is

107

waking up!"

Dr. Bobbitt halted his procedure and spoke to Lester. "Dr. Popkin, I think our patient needs another bolus of fentanyl."

"Right away, Dr. Bobbitt." He infused more fentanyl from a syringe that he hadn't tampered with and the patient quickly went back to sleep. "Sorry, Dr. Bobbitt. Some patients are fast drug metabolizers and need more drugs. I told her not to drink grapefruit juice this morning."

"No problem," Dr. Bobbitt remarked. Lester's explanation as to why Marjorie woke up was a fabrication. Grapefruit juice is known to inhibit liver enzyme activity that would have resulted in more fentanyl being in Marjorie's blood, not less. But Lester needed to cover up his diversion and couldn't think fast enough to make up something that made scientific sense.

The remainder of the transplant operation was completed without further incident. The surgery resident sewed up Marjorie, who was wheeled into the recovery room. Lester walked out of the OR and went directly to the residents' call room without any further comment.

While in the call room, Lester pulled out his diverted drug. Given the events of the day, he felt he'd earned a reward. "Come to papa," he said as he loaded the syringe containing a higher amount of fentanyl than ever before. He hit a vein and pushed the plunger in rapidly and with gusto. Within a few minutes, the lights in the call room went dim. His body went limp and he passed out onto the floor.

The next morning, the surgery and anesthesiology residents started filing into the hospital for their early morning elective procedures. As they were dressing, one of them went to the back of the residents' call room and found Lester lying on the floor. He was dead. The needle of the syringe containing fentanyl was in a vein of his arm. He was still wearing his green operating room scrubs from yesterday.

When it came to Lester Popkin's addiction, Dr. Robert Derksen's mistake was inaction. Maybe it was because he admired him because of his previous athletic talents and gave him the benefit of the doubt. Nevertheless, it was Lester who paid the ultimate price.

*

Fentanyl abuse remains a major source of drug addiction among healthcare workers. Medical specialties that are the most vulnerable to narcotics abuse are anesthesiologists and pharmacists because they have ready access to the drug. The availability of fentanyl patches has created a novel access for abuse. There have been reports of theft of patches that have been taken off of cadavers by autopsy pathologists and their assistants. Systems of checks and double checks have been put in place to minimize abuse. When doctors or nurses are caught abusing drugs, their licenses are revoked by the state licensing boards. To regain a revoked license, a doctor or nurse must enter a physician health rehabilitation program involving regular psychiatric care and twice-a-week random urine drug testing under same-gender witness urine collection. The probation period is typically five years. While this may seem harsh, the program was instituted to protect the health of patients. Impaired physicians are not capable of rational decisions, as clearly seen in Dr. Lester Popkin's case.

I learned about the dangers of fentanyl through the death of Lester Popkin. How can such an intelligent and well-educated man get

109

caught up in this addiction? I thought. Shortly after his death, I was asked to join a physician health program as a toxicology advisor. After serving on the board for many years, I found out that physicians and nurses are very vulnerable populations for drug abuse because of the high stress of their occupations and their easy access to prescription medications.

The Spice of Dyslife

****

Drew Cosgrove knew when he was young that he was different from the other boys in the neighborhood. He never played baseball or football with them. He preferred to hang out with the girls his age on the block. He didn't want to date any of the girls; he wanted to be one of them. They appeared to have more in common with him than the boys. Because he was different growing up, Drew was very shy. He lacked self-confidence and self-worth. His parents knew that he was probably gay or at least headed that way, but they neither encouraged nor discouraged him.

"Drew will just be different from the others," father told mother. Drew's siblings were considerably older siblings, a straight brother who was away at college, and a sister who was married with a child.

As the years passed, some of the girls who were his friends in grade school figured out that Drew was probably gay. Under peer pressure, his old female friends withdrew from him. As a result, Drew was largely alone during his freshman year in high school and was miserable. Trent Monsanto was a school counselor who saw that Drew was struggling to fit in with the other kids. He recognized this in Drew, because he went through something similar when he was young. Trent was a closet homosexual, so nobody at the school knew. He told Drew that he should try out for the after-school theater program. So during his sophomore year, he went for it.

The theater was the best thing that could have happened to Drew. He found his niche as a thespian. He couldn't sing; he couldn't dance; but he found out that he loved to be in front of an audience. He was good at imitating other people's voices and mannerisms, and he could make people laugh. The theater brought him the confidence he never had as a child. His old female playmates saw that he found himself, and were happy for him. They became his friends again. The boys stopped teasing and bullying him like they did throughout grade school. They didn't become his friends, but at least they respected him now.

Some of the other kids in the theater were openly gay. Although the gay boys didn't hit on him, Drew came to the realization that he himself was gay. This actually came as a relief to his parents. At least Drew now knew who he was and could move forward with his life. During his senior year, the school put on the play *One Flew Over the Cuckoo's Nest*. Drew got the lead role. It was sort of fitting, because he felt he hadn't belonged in school just like McMurphy, the character he portrayed, didn't feel he belonged in the asylum. The major difference was that Drew was able to change his environment whereas McMurphy was stuck in his.

Drew went to college, majored in drama, and loved it. He learned about makeup, costumes, set design, props, directing, film editing, casting, and producing. Although acting was his major interest, he thought that if that didn't pan out, he could work behind the scenes. College theater was his opening to pursue acting. His instructors taught him how to immerse himself in a role. He learned how to use facial expressions instead of language. Most of all, he learned that the three most important things to success were: rehearsal, rehearsal, rehearsal. He had to know his lines and everyone else's lines just as if he wrote the play. The most difficult part for him was to visualize how others would see him. So he reviewed video recordings of his rehearsals over and over again. He vowed to himself that no one would outwork him.

Once Drew graduated from college, he moved to Hollywood. His parents, who funded his college expenses, told him that they would support him for two additional years. After that, he was on his own. He had no illusions that Tinseltown would fall in love with him or that there would be many acting parts coming his way. So he got a job cleaning houses. His hours were flexible. This allowed him to schedule appointments and auditions. Drew hired an agent, Jules Cotton. They agreed to change his name. From that point forward, he became Drew Spencer. Over the next five years, Drew Spencer got bit roles in television commercials and supporting acting roles in Community Theater. During one of his shows, Wesley Cable, a manager at a local sporting goods store, saw one of the shows and became enamored with Drew. He went backstage after the show in order to meet the budding actor. There was an immediate connection between the two. Wesley was a large man, nine years older than Drew. After three months, Drew moved into Wesley's apartment. Wesley became very protective of Drew and his young career.

What appeared to be Drew's big break came six months later. His agent got him an audition in a new adaptation of the old Neil Simon play, *The Odd Couple.* He was asked to read the role for Felix Unger, a neat freak. Drew related to this character in real life, as he too had an obsessive-compulsive personality. This trait was especially prominent when he was rehearsing for roles. If he got the part, it would mean steady work for the duration of the run. Drew studied the role played by Jack Lemon in the movie and Tony Randall in the television show. He got a copy of the new script, which he studied intensely.

Drew was preparing for the audition in his apartment. He asked Jules to come over to read the part of Oscar Madison. Wesley was at work at the store. Drew was fidgety and nervous. He knew this was a big moment in his career and didn't want to blow it. Jules sensed that Drew was on edge and wanted to help. He had something that would relax him right in his briefcase. Jules knew that Drew had a sweet tooth and that he kept boxes of cookie mix in the cupboard. He would simply "spice up" this snack in hopes that it would make Drew focus less on his lines and more on letting his natural talent shine through. From his briefcase, Jules pulled out a packet labeled "Spice," which he had just purchased from a local head shop. He emptied the packet into the contents of one of the boxes of cookie mix and baked the mixture in Drew's oven. It would be ready to eat in an hour.

*

As head of the toxicology laboratory, it was part of my job to learn about new poisons circulating through the city where I work. Synthetic cannabinoids such as "Spice" and "K2" are analogs to tetrahydrocannabinol, or THC, the active ingredient in marijuana. In patients with cancer and HIV infections, medical marijuana is used both as an appetite stimulant and suppressor of nausea and vomiting. It was hoped that THC analogs could be made so that they would not be hallucinogenic. One advantage of synthetic cannabis use by abusers is that it is not detected in urine drug screen testing, so individuals can use these cannabinoids without incrimination. Lab identification of synthetic cannabinoids requires more sophisticated techniques, such as mass spectrometry. My toxicology laboratory was able to acquire and test for these cannabinoids. Sometimes I would ask my staff to legally buy them from the places they were sold. Now, when the ER identified a patient suspected of using synthetic cannabis, we had the means to test it. Soon, hospitals across the country were sending urine samples to us.

*

After several hours of frustrating rehearsal, Jules told Drew to take a break. Drew was able to be very convincing as the Felix Unger character, but felt that he wasn't going to get the part unless he improved. Jules brought out the laced cookies, hoping to improve Drew's attitude. After they each had two cookies, and were relaxing for a few minutes, Jules got a phone call. It was another client of his who needed to discuss a contract. "Drew, I have to meet someone, but when I return, let's go over the second scene." Jules put on his jacket and left.

Drew was still seated on the sofa when he became light-headed, dizzy, agitated, and even more anxious than before; it had nothing to do with the upcoming audition. He called Wesley at his office.

"What's the matter, Drew?"

"I was rehearsing with Jules and I suddenly got nauseous. I feel like I'm high but it's different than before," he told Wesley.

"Where is Jules?"

"He had to leave. Wesley, I really feel weird. Things are spinning in my head."

Their apartment was on the fifth floor. "Don't go anywhere Drew. I'll be right there." Wesley grabbed his coat, told his co-workers at the store that there was an emergency and he drove home.

Drew was still lying down on the sofa when Wesley arrived. "How do you feel now?" Wesley asked.

"Still crappy."

Wesley got Drew off the sofa, took him by the hand, and led him into the bedroom. He took off Drew's shoes and socks, and put him into bed underneath the bed covers. Wesley turned off the light, closed the bedroom door and went to the kitchen to make some coffee. Maybe that would settle his nerves. He sat down for a few minutes and all was calm. Then he heard a commotion in the bedroom. Wesley got up from the kitchen table to see if Drew needed something. When he opened the bedroom door, he got the shock of his life. Drew either jumped or fell out of the window. There was a swimming pool directly under the apartment. But the pool was covered and it contained only a few feet of water. Not enough to break Drew's fall. Wesley poked his head outside the window and saw that Drew was face down on the pool cover, not moving. Wesley frantically ran out of the apartment, raced down the stairs and out the main door. Some people who were walking by gathered outside. Wesley screamed to one of them.

"For god's sake, call an ambulance! Call 9-1-1." Wesley

picked up Drew's limp body. Drew was alive but unconscious. Wesley took off his shirt and covered Drew's upper body in an attempt to keep him warm.

"Where is that ambulance?" he said to no one in particular. A few minutes later, he heard the sirens. It was the longest nine minutes of his life. The paramedics arrived and gently transferred Drew to their gurney and into the ambulance. Wesley joined them in the ambulance and they drove off. They went to the hospital where all the Hollywood stars go. But this was not how Drew wanted his name to be connected with other actors.

Drew suffered massive injuries to his legs and hips and had extensive internal bleeding. He was listed in critical condition. Wesley waited nervously outside the OR. When Drew's vital signs stabilized, he was moved into intensive care. Blood and urine was sent to the clinical laboratory for analysis. There was no alcohol or recreational drugs detected in any of the lab's drug screens.

Jules returned to Drew's apartment and saw that there were police all around the building. He asked what happened and the cops told him that someone fell out the window of the apartment. Jules looked up and saw the broken window. He couldn't be certain, but he thought it was Drew's bedroom window. Upon hearing that, Jules ran into the building and headed up to the apartment. When he arrived, there was yellow tape around the front door that read, "CRIME SCENE DO NOT CROSS." He then thought to himself, *was it Drew who fell out the window?*

One of the policemen asked Jules to identify himself.

Jules responded, "Drew is an actor and I am his agent. He was rehearsing lines for an audition this evening. He was fine when I left to see someone." Jules then saw that one of the detectives was looking at the uneaten cookies in the kitchen. Jules' heart sank. *Could the marijuana in the cookies have caused this?* he asked himself. The policeman asked about the cookies and Jules acknowledged that he had baked them. But he didn't tell him about the synthetic marijuana. The empty Spice package was still in his pocket.

Maybe they won't find out about it. But then he saw the detective put the cookies into a bag labeled "Evidence. Crime Scene." He told the other detective that he was going to have the crime lab analyze them for hallucinogens. At that point, Jules broke down and admitted to having adulterated the cookies.

"It's all my fault. I laced the cookies with marijuana. But I didn't think there would be this accident, for god's sake." Jules was taken into custody and held over in the police station pending further investigation.

Over the next few hours, Drew's medical condition worsened. Wesley was nearby the entire time. Drew never opened his eyes or regained consciousness. Early in the morning of the next day, he passed away. The cause of death was listed as injuries incurred from a fall. Postmortem blood and tissue samples were sent to my lab for synthetic marijuana analysis. Some of the cookies Drew ate were also sent. Using mass spectrometry, we confirmed the presence of Spice in the cookie and blood samples. This information was used to charge Jules with involuntary manslaughter. He had no motive to harm Drew, and the drugs that he'd spiked the cookies with were legal in the

U.S. at the time, so Jules was acquitted of all charges.

*

Synthetic cannabinoids were originally synthesized by John W. Huffman, an organic chemistry professor at Clemson University. Dr. Huffman tried to find chemical substitutes for delta-9-tetrahydrocannabinol or THC, the active ingredient in marijuana. Despite the original honorable intent, synthetic cannabinoids are now being sold as recreational drugs. They are labeled with names like Spice, K2, and Fire and Ice. Dr. Huffman synthesized hundreds of synthetic cannabinoids; many of them are labeled with a number and with his initials, JWH. Drug standards that are needed for mass spectrometric analysis are not commercially available for all of the synthetic THC that he produced. Workplace drug testing programs have not included testing for synthetic cannabis among federal employees. Therefore, Spice and K2 remain a means for getting high while escaping detection.

In 2012, following a surge of emergency room cases involving patients who used synthetic bath salts containing mephedrone and synthetic cannabis, such as JWH-18, many states enacted legislation banning the sale and distribution of these drugs. The U.S. Drug Enforcement Agency used their right of emergency legislation to list 5 synthetic marijuana substitutes on their Schedule I of Controlled Substances. Unfortunately, this has led to the private manufacture of second-generation synthetic drugs. A more prudent act, which some states have initiated, would be to ban all synthetic cannabinoids so that any drug analog that produces similar physiologic effects would be illegal. It is ironic that in California, where marijuana use is highly prevalent, the use of synthetic cannabinoids lags behind most of the other states. It is likely an economic issue of supply and demand. The high availability of true marijuana at lower costs than Spice reduces demand for the synthetic

119

versions.   A similar situation may now exist in Washington and Colorado, where marijuana is now legal.

Rave Review

Even though this was an annual event, it took nearly an entire year of planning for the next rave party to be held in the city. Last year, more than 3,000 teenagers and young adults came to hear fast-paced electronic music in the "techno" and "psytrance" genres. There was a combination of live performances and disk jockeys. The arena was equipped with elaborate sound equipment; sophisticated computer-controlled lighting, including strobes synchronized to the music; and artificial smoke that filled the air. Kids came from all over the state with their lasers and glow sticks to dance, socialize, and soak up the scene.

"Each year, this just gets better and better," was a quote from one of the ravers. Paul Fiona was head of the Rave Planning Committee. There were thousands of minute details that needed to be addressed. These included commercial sponsorship, getting the appropriate permits from the city, contacting the media, ticketing, food, advertisement, merchandising, staffing, volunteers, lighting, audio equipment, venue issues, even Porta-Potty rentals since there was always a backup in the women's restrooms. The bands themselves were organized by a separate committee. Some of the better-known groups required special attention, including the handling of all local transportation, hotel accommodations, food, and drinks. Paul assigned a local host to each band. The host would stay with each group during their tour and attend to all of their needs.

A medical unit was established inside the venue with signage alerting to its existence. Since most of the attendees were young, Paul had few concerns that there would be any serious cardiac events. But he knew that it got very warm inside the arena, especially in the mosh pit at the center of the arena where kids are tightly packed and are all dancing together. Attendees had fainted in past years. Security was a major issue. He hired retired cops and private security companies to make sure that there wasn't any unruly behavior. Their duties included traffic control and parking. Paul scheduled extra people to be on hand after the event. In the past, this was when most of the trouble occurred. Fire safety was a top priority for Paul. He studied the Providence, Rhode Island fire of 2007, where exits were blocked and pyrotechnics were allowed. Most of the attendees died in the fire because they couldn't get out fast enough. This was not going to happen here, not on Paul's watch. No smoking, fireworks, or pyrotechnics were allowed. He put up extra signs pointing out the exits, and ensured that none of them were blocked. He also assigned people to man each entrance so no one would be able to sneak in.

The date of the big event was drawing near. Paul trusted that everything was in order and that the event would be a success. This was the first concert of this magnitude he'd ever been in charge of. He knew that if he put on a great show, there would be more demand for his services as an event planner. He thought he had everything covered. Paul knew that many of the partygoers would be using Ecstasy. Nobody had any really serious problems before. But he couldn't anticipate everything.

*

Fredrick Samuels was known on the street as "Smooth Dog." He had been a drug pusher ever since high school. He came from a broken family and knew from the beginning that there was only one person who would look out for him, and that was himself. Smooth started out pushing pot, but later got involved with crack, meth, and Ecstasy. He had been arrested a few times. But each time, he got a little smarter about the business and not getting caught. Now, he hired people who did the actual sales and distribution. He got quality product from a local, clandestine laboratory and put his own special logo on the drugs. In this way, repeat users could ask for a specific supply by name. Smooth got a special Ecstasy batch just for the upcoming rave party. The supplier said it was some of the best stuff they'd ever made. Smooth stamped on his special logo. It read, "Prime." He instructed his team to give out free samples to the partygoers in order to get them hooked.

"Tell them, that it's the beat, the music, and the flashing lights along with the Ecstasy that makes it a real trip," he instructed his employees. "So go out and make old Smoothie proud."

*

Alicia Cheng worked as a store clerk at a local grocery store since her junior year in high school. Her family didn't have the money to send her to college, nor was she inclined to go. Alicia heard about the rave from her friends who went last year. She was not naïve about Ecstasy. She tried it at some other parties and really liked it. It relaxed her and made her feel more compassionate toward her friends than she was normally. Sometimes the next day she would feel a little down, but it was worth it to her. So when a group of her friends asked her to go to the rave party, she didn't turn them down. She and three of her girlfriends drove to the event and had a tailgate party in the parking lot an hour before the event opened. One of them brought a case of beer to get everyone loosened up. When the doors finally opened, she and her friends piled out of the van and into the arena. They brought pacifiers, stuffed animals, and gloves with LED lights on them. Ecstasy promotes nurturing and emotional feelings in users, and these props perpetuate these illusions. Alicia brought a stuffed panda bear.

Smooth distributed his agents throughout the arena. They were hitting on anyone who looked like an Ecstasy buyer. One of his sellers, Jonesy, came across Alicia and her gang. "Hey girls are you here to have fun tonight?" he teased them.

"You know it," one of them said back to him. They all knew why Jonesy was there and what he was selling.

So one of Alicia's friends was about to slip Jonesy a ten-dollar bill when he surprised them all and said, "The first one is on me, pretty one." He handed each of them a pill. "Plenty more where this comes from. Remember the brand," he said as he moved on. The girls went to the bathroom, and with their water bottles in hand, they each swallowed a pill. Alicia stuffed the empty envelope into her pocket as she left the bathroom.

The concert was just getting started when Alicia started to feel funny. She was not getting the usual effects of the drug. Instead of relaxation, she felt tense. Instead of warmth, she felt chills. Instead of empathy, she felt paranoia. "Get away from me," she said to her friends, who were looking at her strangely. The lights, the loud music, the warm temperatures, the hot sweaty bodies all around her made her panic. She rushed to get out for some fresh air. Her breathing and heart started racing. Her mouth was extremely dry. She started sweating profusely.

I can't see where I'm going, she said to herself. *Everything's a blur.* Suddenly, she passed out. She hit her head on the hard floor of the arena. At first, nobody saw her fall, as it was dark and everyone was into their own thing. She had separated herself from her friends. After a few minutes, someone noticed a girl down and tried to help her up. But she was unresponsive. A group of people carried her out to behind the stadium area. Her panda fell onto the floor and was trampled by ravers. Someone went to the medic station for help. The paramedics tried to revive her without success. Paul had arranged to have an ambulance stationed at the arena during the entire show. Alicia was put onto a gurney, loaded into the ambulance and headed off to the General Hospital. A call was placed to the emergency department alerting the ED staff of an incoming patient.

A television reporter covering the party saw what was happening to Alicia. Marvin Scott called his editor about a breaking story and the station instructed a camera team to head over to the General Hospital. The cameramen packed their equipment that was originally set up to film the stage shows. Marvin couldn't wait for the crew to finish, so he jumped into his car and followed the ambulance en route to the hospital.

While being transported in the ambulance, Alicia began seizing. The paramedics did the best they could to prevent her from harming herself and swallowing her tongue. When they arrived at the hospital, Alicia was immediately evaluated by the emergency department team. She was unconscious and had a very low Glascow Coma Score. The GSC is a widely used and objective measure of an individual's consciousness. A fully awake person has a score of 15, while the minimum score is for someone in a deep coma. The ED staff recorded Alicia's score; it was a three, the lowest on the scale. Alicia was extremely warm, with a body temperature of 103°F. She received IV fluids and was transferred to the medical intensive care unit. Once there, a cooling protocol was initiated by the staff. A Foley catheter was inserted and a urine sample was sent to the lab. It came back 40 minutes later as positive for Ecstasy. There were no other drugs detected in her system. Ecstasy alone should not have caused this serious problem.

News reporters, including Marvin Scott, gathered outside the hospital, wanting to know what happened and how Alicia was doing. Police officers were also on the scene hoping to interview Alicia or her friends. Updates interrupted local broadcasting throughout the evening. This resulted in hundreds of telephone calls to the local TV and radio stations, and to the General Hospital itself, from anxious parents whose sons and daughters were still at the rave. Most of the attendees didn't know what was happening and couldn't hear their cell phones or had them turned off due to the loud music. Marvin discovered that five other ravers suffered effects similar to Alicia's, but in varying degrees of severity. They were sent to other hospitals for treatment. Interestingly, all of those affected were of Indian descent.

I got paged at my home that night shortly after Alicia was admitted to the emergency department. The clinical toxicologist from the Poison Control Center, Dr. Jean Murphy, who was consulted on the case, contacted Dr. Ray Gervais, one of my analytical toxicologists, to see if my lab could determine if Alicia overdosed on methylenedioxyethylamphetamine, or MDMA, the active drug in Ecstasy, or if there was a contaminant in the drug that was causing her problems.

The police were also interested in the answer to this question because it might determine how they would proceed with a criminal investigation. They'd heard from other partygoers that there was someone giving Ecstasy pills away for free. So they obtained some of the drugs, and delivered an assortment of Ecstasy pills to the lab at the General Hospital for Ray to conduct his analysis. In the meantime, the police asked that someone from the emergency department search Alicia's possessions. In the pocket of her jeans, they found the pill packet with "Prime" stamped on the outside. The empty packet was also sent to the lab for testing. Ray knew that trace amounts of the drug might still be present, which could provide the link between the drug and what was found in Alicia's blood and urine.

Ray worked through the night hoping to get some results for the intensive care unit team that might help Alicia. During a break in his work, he went up to the unit to see her. Alicia's family was in the waiting room next door. A woman, whom he presumed to be her mother, was crying uncontrollably. Ray walked past the waiting room without making eye contact, and headed straight toward the main ICU door. He flashed his hospital identification card and the guard let him in. Alicia was

127

covered in a cooling blanket. She had a breathing tube inserted through her mouth, and tubing connecting IVs to the veins in her arm. There were also arterial catheters in her arm for drawing blood for analysis of oxygen, carbon dioxide and acid-base balance. Her eyes were taped closed. Jean Murphy saw Ray come in and waved him over.

"How's she doing?" Ray asked.

Dr. Murphy responded, "Not well. She has significant internal bleeding. The next few hours will be critical. Have you found out anything yet on the toxicology tests?"

"I've extracted the drugs as well as Alicia's blood and urine, and they've been injected into our mass spectrometer. We'll know in 30 minutes." With that, Ray left the ICU, even more committed to learning the truth about what happened to Alicia.

When he returned to the lab, he looked at the mass spectrometer data. At the General, my group developed novel toxicology strategies based on high-resolution mass spectrometry. Rather than bombarding drugs to produce fragments whose masses must be matched against standardized libraries, our high-resolution technique enables detection of the exact mass of any unaltered compounds found in a sample, i.e., without mass fragmentation. This information can then be used to determine the molecular formula of the compound. In this way, the database from which unknowns can be identified is greatly expanded. A chemical structure simply can be typed into an Internet search program, and a listing of matching compounds appears. "You can more readily tell what something is from looking at the whole puzzle rather than trying to figure it out from the individual pieces," I told my students.

Ray looked at the results from Alicia's blood and urine, and the various pills of Ecstasy recovered at the party. He was particularly interested in the pill labeled "Prime." The toxicology data clearly showed the presence of Ecstasy in all of Alicia's samples and also in the pills. The concentration was higher in her system than expected for a single ingestion. When he looked at the concentration contained within the Prime pill itself, he found that the amount present was five times the amount typically produced by labs. Smooth unknowingly overdosed Alicia and the others who were stricken. Ray was not able to identify any contaminants in any of the samples he tested. It was strictly an overdose situation. I concurred with Ray's conclusion and we paged Dr. Murphy to tell her of our findings. This information was relayed to the hospitals that were treating the other Ecstasy toxicity cases.

Meanwhile, Alicia's medical course was deteriorating. She developed multi-organ failure, including liver and kidney failure, cardiac arrest, and a bleeding disorder. The team initiated a massive transfusion protocol due to Alicia's bleeding. A decision was made by the medical team to try continuous veno-venous hemofiltration on Alicia even before they learned from Ray that she indeed had an overdose of Ecstasy. This is a specialized dialysis procedure that is targeted toward the removal of low molecular weight toxins. Despite these efforts, they could not rescue Alicia, and she expired about five hours after her arrival at the emergency department. Ray was present when the news was released to the family. It was not a pleasant scene for Ray, who had never been confronted by the death of a young person before. Everyone on Alicia's medical team was touched by her death. Ray was not much comforted by the fact that he knew he did everything he could.

None of the other cases from the rave party resulted in a fatality. My team was curious as to why the Ecstasy poisoning cases only occurred in those of Indian heritage. We planned to conduct a genetic correlation study to see if we could identify a specific gene or mutation present in high frequency among Indians, which would have made Alicia and the others genetically susceptible to the adverse effects of the drug. Unfortunately, due to privacy laws, we were able to get permission to obtain DNA from just two of the other Ecstasy patients who got sick at the rave. In some hospitals, patients are asked to sign a statement that gives researchers permission to use blood specimens for future medical purposes if the identity of these samples is permanently removed. The hospitals in our region do not ask for such permission.

The police concluded that all of the rave partygoers who got sick had taken Prime. After interviewing a number of people, they were able to identify that Smooth Dog provided the drugs to Jonesy. They were both located and promptly arrested. They were charged with voluntary manslaughter and endangerment to a minor. Paul Fiona's big event turned out to be the worst nightmare he could have ever imagined. While no one blamed him for the unfortunate occurrences at the rave, he was forever associated with this tragedy. He left his once promising career as an event planner and found something else to do with his life.

*

Rave parties continue to occur throughout the United States, Europe, and the Far East. Law enforcement agencies have been powerless to prevent these gatherings. Young undercover cops do their best to catch and arrest pushers in the act of distributing during concerts. After the death of Alicia Cheng, a city councilman introduced legislation to ban concerts held on public property that promote an environment conducive to Ecstasy use. Unfortunately, the action was viewed as a violation of individual rights for free speech and expression. "You cannot ban a style of music," the opponents argued. In Los Angeles, a fifteen-year old girl recently died of respiratory arrest and multi-organ failure caused by an Ecstasy overdose. Her mother was interviewed on local television. "I was supposed to be planning her Sweet Sixteen party," she said. "Now I have to plan her funeral."

Pooper Scooper

****

Ronald Brown was a career Navy man. He joined immediately after high school and became seaman first class after basic training. He served on a destroyer, an aircraft carrier, and his last assignment was the USS Santa Cruz, a missile cruiser. Ronny got a sailor's tattoo on his large bicep decades before it became fashionable for everyone else to have tats. It featured a large anchor and the letters "USN." Ronny rose through the ranks and eventually became the chief petty officer. He was one of the first African Americans in U.S. history to receive this appointment. By then, he was in his late forties. Although some white sailors initially had a problem with his authority, Chief Brown treated everyone fairly, and the prejudice was quickly dispelled. He respected the officers and enjoyed his role as a leader and mentor to the other enlisted men. Ronny was a tough guy but he tried not to show it. When he was younger, he once competed in the U.S. Armed Forces Boxing Tournament. As a middleweight, he got to the third round before losing to a guy who eventually went pro. Ronny's boxing career was short lived; he developed problems with his shoulder and retired from the ring.

Ronny was not married. Like many of the other guys, he would sometimes visit brothels in the ports of call where his ship was docked. One particularly popular establishment was the

"Tender Trap." Unlike other sailors who wanted a variety of kinky sex, Ronny would almost always do it in the missionary position. He usually chose a girl who could speak at least some broken English. The USS Santa Cruz was stationed in the Gulf of Thailand for many months, near but not directly in North Korean waters. If there were any hostilities they could be on the scene in a matter of hours. When he was on shore leave in Bangkok, Ronny began seeing one girl in particular.

*

Tamarine was born to a poor family. Tamarine was five and her sister Kamala was six when their father, who was a dock-worker, was asked to join a merchant ship as a deckhand. He never returned. Their mother was a cook at a local restaurant in the port. She worked hard each day and tried her best to raise her daughters. But they both became prostitutes by the time they were in their early teenage years. Most of their clients were seamen visiting the harbor. The girls were given housing, food, and minimal medical care, but little else. There was no attempt made by the bordello to educate them. Tamarine, Kamala, and the other girls had a grim future, but there was little they could do about it. Tamarine saw that when the older girls lost their looks, they were cast onto the streets. By then, many of these girls were addicted to cocaine or opium. Tamarine was prettier than Kamala and therefore attracted more customers. She was also smarter than most of the girls, and despite any formal training, she picked up quite a bit of English from the sailors.

Ronny first met Tamarine when he picked her out of a line-up of girls at the Tender Trap. By then, Tamarine had been there three years and was a veteran in the business. She used a lot of makeup to make her even more attractive. She knew how to sway her hips to entice the servicemen. It was all about making them happy while earning money for herself and her sister. Someday, they would leave this awful place. At first, Ronny saw her as just one of the other hookers, only younger. But as the evening went on, he found himself more than just physically attracted to her, even though he was more than 30 years her senior. When he returned to the ship, he couldn't stop thinking about her sweet face and innocent smile. During his next shore leave, he headed straight for the Tender Trap and asked for Tamarine by name. He was happy that she was available and was not with another man. As time went on, their encounters were less about sex and more about companionship. Her English improved and she was able to carry on a conversation. He started asking her about her life, how she came to work at the brothel, and what she did when she was not with a john.

She, in turn, asked Ronny how life was on the USS Santa Cruz. Ronny told Tamerine that the job was getting tedious. He was thinking of retiring from the service and settling down back home. The madam at the Tender Trap saw that there was a connection being made between Ronny and Tamarine, but did nothing to discourage it. Ronny tipped well and never caused any trouble.

After about eight months, Ronny went into Captain Craig Lohman's quarters to discuss Ronny's discharge from the Navy. He was entitled to a good pension and lifetime medical care. At 48, he was still young enough to start another career. Ronny served with Captain Lohman for nearly nine years and had a good rapport with him. The captain laid out the retirement procedure and paperwork; within a month, Ronny would be a civilian for the first time since he was a teenager. The captain asked Ronny where he wanted his port of exit. When he said "Bangkok," the captain knew that there was somebody waiting for him there.

Ronny asked Tamarine to marry him and leave Thailand for America. He had to first pay the madam of the Tender Trap for the loss of her "employee." Tamarine gladly accepted Ronny's marriage proposal. Most of the other girls were happy for her and threw her a small party. Her sister Kamala was sad because she was going to be left behind. Tamarine promised her that when they were established in the States and had some extra money, they would return to get her. Kamala had a premonition that she would never see her sister again.

Ronny found out that for immigration purposes, it would be better for him to wed Tamarine under U.S. jurisdiction than in Thailand. So he asked his captain for one last favor, a privilege he thought his superior officer had as captain of a Navy vessel.

"Actually, sea captains do not have the authority to marry seamen or anyone else," Captain Lohman told Ronny. "But I happened to also be an ordained minister, so I can do this for you." After a week, it was all arranged. The boat was decked out for the retiring CPO. A makeshift altar was created. Kamala and the sisters' mother attended.

"Do you Tamarine Janpong take Chief Petty Officer, um I mean, Citizen Ronald Brown to be your lawfully wedded husband?"

"I am," she said quickly, in case the offer got rescinded.

136

Then realizing her mistake, she said, "No, I mean I do!"

The captain repeated the question to Ronny. After his answer, Captain Lohman concluded, "By the power vested in me by the State of California, I now pronounce you, husband and wife. You may kiss the bride." The USS Santa Cruz Marine Corp Band played the Wedding March, and Tamarine and Ronny walked under an arch of swords of the ship's Sword Detail. The blades were unsheathed pair-by-pair and the swords rotated so that the blades faced away from the couple as they passed under. Tamarine became Mrs. Ronald Brown. They honeymooned in Singapore and flew to the States two weeks later to start their new life.

*

Tamarine and Ronny decided to move to the San Diego area where they rented an apartment near Ocean Beach. This area reminded Tamarine of Bangkok. Lots of sailors and ex-sailors lived there, so it also was very comfortable for Ronny. Ronny applied for a job at a bar that was owned by one of the officers he had served. Lieutenant John Dank served 10 years in the Navy but never wanted to be a career man. When he retired, he opened up a saloon called Last Call. At first, Ronny worked as a bouncer. His toughness helped deter any fights. But Ronny didn't want to just be the muscle. So he went to school to train as a bartender. Dank was more than happy to give Ronny a bartending job and a raise when he'd completed his training.

Life in the States was much more of an adjustment for Tamarine. Although there were a lot of Asians living in the area, she didn't know anyone other than Ronny, and there were very few people who spoke her language. She began to feel very isolated. She missed Kamala. Shortly after her arrival in the States, Tamarine found out that her mother died of food poisoning, which made her even sadder than she already was. She didn't have any working skills other than "escort services," which Ronny naturally forbade. She'd left that world when she came to America. So she got a job as a maid at a nearby hotel. She didn't have a car so she walked to work. She begged Ronny to allow her to get pregnant. A baby would give her something to care for, she reasoned. Ronny was not hot on the idea, as he was almost fifty.

He told John Dank, "I'll be pushing up the daisies by the time this kid is in high school." But Ronny relented and Tamarine quickly got pregnant. During her prenatal visits, she disclosed that she used to work in a brothel. She had a history of syphilis infection and hepatitis A, but no active disease. She was negative for laboratory tests for human immunodeficiency virus, hepatitis B and C, and gonorrhea.

Tamarine gave birth to her baby in the spring of the following year. The baby was five weeks early and weighed 4 pounds 7 ounces. Ronny waited in the maternity ward lounge rather than join Tamarine in the delivery room to witness the birth; his generation of men didn't do that sort of thing. Other than its prematurity, the baby girl appeared healthy. The child was named Isra, which meant "nocturnal journey" in Arabic; Ronny and Tamarine felt it was appropriate given Tamarine's own travels through her short life.

While baby Isra was still in the hospital, a sample of her meconium was scooped into a specimen cup and sent to the clinical laboratory to test for the presence of recreational drugs.

Meconium is the *in utero* feces that is initially formed during the third and fourth months of pregnancy and remains in the gastrointestinal tract of the fetus until delivery. A dark sticky material that is very different from normal stools, meconium is normally excreted from the baby at the time of birth or shortly thereafter. Some of Tamarine's urine was also collected and sent to the lab for drug testing. This was an acceptable practice to rule out drug abuse as a cause of low birth weight infants. Both of these tests were conducted without Tamarine or Ronny's knowledge or permission. Tamarine's urine turned out to be completely negative for any recreational drugs. However, Isra's meconium was positive for cocaine. Recreational drugs taken by the mother during pregnancy accumulate in the meconium. Children of crack cocaine mothers have developmental delays and learning disabilities. While a positive urine drug test indicates drug use within a few days of delivery, a positive result in meconium indicates more regular use throughout the pregnancy. Thus, a negative urine drug test result does not contradict a positive meconium finding. It can be interpreted as drug abstinence just prior to delivery. The results were relayed to the pediatrician, who contacted the Office of Child Protective Services. There would be a review of the adequacy of Tamarine and Ronald to care for the child.

The initial test was conducted by the laboratory using a drug screening methodology. Protective Services asked the laboratory to have the result sent out for confirmation drug testing. My lab has been conducting meconium testing for many years for babies delivered at the General Hospital. Since my hospital is an indigent facility that serves the underprivileged and uninsured, many of the women who deliver their babies are known users of crack cocaine, heroin, or methamphetamines. These mothers are not able to care for their children financially, emotionally, or psychologically. Positive drug testing from my laboratory sometimes leads to the removal of the child from its home and into foster care. But very few of these cases are contested by the affected mother or family members, if there is a family. Most of these mothers return to the streets to hook and continue to abuse drugs. Nevertheless, I had to be sure my analytical data was forensically defensible in case there was a legal challenge. So in addition to the screening test that many hospitals are doing, we also developed a confirmatory test based on mass spectrometry. Word got out within the clinical toxicology community that we offer this confirmatory procedure, and many other hospital laboratories sent us meconium for testing. Isra's meconium was received at the General Hospital and tested positive for benzoylecgonine, a principal metabolite of cocaine.

Armed with my laboratory report, Protective Services convened a hearing to determine the suitability of Tamarine and Ronny as Isra's parents. Protective Services learned that Tamarine was a former prostitute and her sexually transmitted disease history was uncovered. Ronny was much older than her. If she was an unfit mother, would he be around and be able to care for the child? His income was modest, which was also a factor. The fact that they were a racially mixed couple may have played a role in the committee's opinion, although this argument was not stated, as it was clearly discriminatory.

When Ronny found out that Isra's meconium was

positive with cocaine, he immediately confronted Tamarine.

"Where are you getting this drug? I brought you all the way from Thailand and this is how you treat me? How could you do this to me?"

Tamarine pleaded her innocence to Ronny. "I not do this," she said in her broken English. "I know girls used coke back home, but not sister or me. I a good girl."

Ronny searched the house for any evidence of free base or crack cocaine use. He found no papers, powders, razors, pipes, or even matches. One of his Navy friends told him that there was a way to check for cocaine dust. These kits were intended for parents as a means for checking up on their kids. So he bought a kit through the Internet, swiped Tamarine's dresser and bathroom and sent it off to a laboratory for cocaine testing. The results were negative for any drugs. Ronny was then convinced his wife was innocent.

During the hearing, the committee's psychiatrists conducted separate interviews with Tamarine and Ronny. Tamarine's command of English was a problem as she misinterpreted some of the questions. Ronny admitted to the committee that he was not initially in favor of having children, but stated that his opinion changed once he saw and held Isra. They asked if he would have preferred a boy, and although he said no, his body language said otherwise. Tamarine was asked if she was still selling herself behind Ronny's back to the local sailors to make money. She completely denied this, saying that this was in her past. She did say her sister was still a Bangkok prostitute, which didn't help her case. All things considered, Protective Services ruled against the Brown family and they took

Isra away. Tamarine cried uncontrollably as Ronny escorted her out of the hearing room.

Ronny vowed to fight back. He hired a former officer who had served with him on the USS Santa Cruz who was now a lawyer in the area. Sam Garcia thought there may have been some racial profiling in the Brown's case. Garcia in turn, contacted me to find out more about the drug testing we conducted. "Once we receive a sample in the lab," I explained, "we have tight security as to where it has been and where it is kept. Everyone who is involved with the specimen is documented with signatures, dates, and times. We pay particular attention to the integrity of the seal, and reject any sample if the seal is broken before we get to it." I showed him the chain-of-custody paperwork that documented every step of the process. Sam could find no fault with our lab's documentation.

But then I remarked, "In my experience, the documentation of specimen custody at the hospital where the meconium is taken is often lacking. In the newborn wards, there are babies crying, there are mothers, family members, doctors, residents, interns, nurses, social workers, and aides who are constantly coming and going. It can be very chaotic. I suggest you check the documentation of the meconium orders itself."

Sam returned to the hospital and ordered all the medical records and progress notes on Tamarine's delivery. The hospital did not have an electronic order entry system. Sam tried to trace the steps that led to the ordering of meconium testing on Tamarine. In Isra's progress notes, there was no mention of the need to order a meconium test. It was unclear who exactly ordered the test. The laboratory and pharmacy order sheet was also devoid of a specific request. Sam went to the laboratory and retrieved the original paper requisition laboratory slip that accompanied the specimen. While the time and date of when the specimen was received in the lab were stamped, there was no physician's name listed. Sam noticed that the date and time of the sample was a Saturday evening. No other lab tests were ordered on Isra's blood or urine within four hours of the time stamp. I told Sam that laboratory errors occurred more often on weekends and holidays when there were fewer staff on hand, and more part-time employees working.

Referring to birthdates, I told Mr. Garcia, "You can't ask Mother Nature to adhere to our workday schedule." Sam asked to see the records of the other babies present in the ward that day. He found that the ward was completely filled. He was able to determine that the urine of another mother, who delivered on the same day as Tamarine, was positive for cocaine. While there was a request for meconium testing of that baby, the lab did not receive a sample for testing. Could there have been a sample mix-up? Was Isra's meconium really that from this other child? Sam requested that the Child Protective Services reconvene to hear the latest evidence.

Given the poor documentation of the meconium test request, Child Protective Services rescind their decision. Isra was returned to her parents. Protective Services tendered no letter of apology or admission of guilt. They made Tamarine and Ronny feel that they were lucky to get their baby back based on a technicality. Isra lived at the foster home for six months. As per policy, there were no visitation rights granted to Tamarine and Ronny during that time. By all accounts, Isra was a normal and healthy baby. Tamarine now hugged her baby and told her she would never let her go. Isra cooed and smiled. She seemed to know that Tamarine was her mother.

Sam Garcia filed suit against the hospital on behalf of Ronny and Tamarine. Not wanting any bad publicity, the hospital settled the suit. The terms included no admission of guilt. Tamarine didn't care; she had Isra back. With the settlement money, Tamarine arranged to have her sister stop working at the Tender Trap and move to San Diego. Tamarine and Ronny met Kamala at the airport upon her arrival. Little Isra was there too. Their reunion resulted in more tears. This time, they were tears of joy.

*

The National Institute on Drug Abuse has determined that in 2008, 16% of girls between 15 and 17 years old used illicit drugs during pregnancy, compared with 7% illicit drug use for pregnant women between 18 and 25, and 2% illicit drug use for pregnant women between 26 and 44. The corresponding rate for binge alcohol use for these same age groups of pregnant girls and women was 14%, 5%, and 4%, respectively. Meconium testing for drugs of abuse is a common practice at hospitals that serve a population rife with drug abusers. These tests cannot be used to determine in utero alcohol exposure.

Computerized order entry systems and electronic medical records are becoming the standard for the medical industry. In most hospitals today, a test cannot be ordered unless it comes directly from a qualified physician or staff member. In Tamarine's case, a computerized record would have required there to be documentation from the ordering physician. The program would not have allowed sample submission without this part being completed. Sample mix-ups have been significantly reduced as the result of implementing these systems.

Pressor Luck

****

Deidre Murphy had one, and only one objective for going to nursing school. She wanted to meet and marry a doctor so that she could live the lifestyle of a doctor's wife. There would be country club memberships, social events, bridge clubs, and hobnobbing with the rich and famous. She would have a maid, gardener, and chauffeur; her kids would have nannies and they would go to private schools. Deidre came from a working-class family. Her mother worked as a waitress for 20 years. She resented her mother for the life she had as a child. She vowed that her own life would be different. So all through high school, she only dated boys who looked as if they were going places. Not the ones who were poor like her and headed nowhere. Deidre was attractive but not a knockout. She made the most of her appearance with makeup and hairstyle. She tried not to look too slutty, but provocative enough to attract attention. Unfortunately, her plan for the most part was a washout. When the boys she was targeting found out she came from the wrong side of the tracks, they didn't give her a second look. It was then that she decided on nursing school. Deidre worked for two years as a waitress to save enough money to go to nursing school. Her grades were fine. It was just a matter of getting financial aid since her family didn't have the means to support her education

Once in nursing school, Deidre was an above-average student. She did well on her written and practical exams, though at times, she cheated on multiple-choice tests by looking over the shoulder of one of the smarter students when the test monitor wasn't looking. She also hated the work itself. The idea of having to serve the needs of others was disgusting to her.

I should be the one being waited on hand and foot, she thought to herself. But what motivated her to continue was the belief that this was her only meal ticket to a better life. So when she graduated, she interned at the General Hospital in the Intensive Care Unit. Most of these patients were not awake or intubated and unable to speak. This was the perfect job placement for her.

It's bad enough that I have to nurse them, I don't want to have to chitchat with them about their stupid problems too, she thought. Despite her negative attitude, she didn't show any of it in her interactions with the patients, her superiors, or the other nurses on the floor. When it came to the ICU residents, she was particularly attentive and interactive.

Deidre did well enough that she was hired as an ICU nurse. At the time, there was a nursing shortage so this job was not difficult for her to get. Many ICU nurses burn out after a few years because of the high stress of the job. The nurses in the oncology wards have similarly high rates of turnover. Deidre never had this problem. She didn't care about her patients, and to her, they were nothing more than slabs of meat. Her true objectives were the young interns who were training at the hospital, who would one day be rich and successful doctors.

Deidre was successful in attracting the attention of

several of the better-looking male doctors for sex after hours. Unfortunately, most of them were married and these affairs didn't last long. Deidre often thought of calling one of the wives after a breakup to get even, but resisted the temptation. If word got out that she was "kissing and telling," it would ruin her chances of any success in the future.

The ICU at the General was organized into five separate units. The coronary care unit treated cardiac patients, the surgical unit saw patients after elective and emergency surgery, the NICU tended to neonates who were born prematurely, the pediatric ICU treated children and teenagers, and the medical intensive care unit, where Deidre was assigned, cared for mostly elderly patients that were sent from nursing homes for acute care. Occasionally they would die while in the unit, often of heart failure. The MICU consisted of eight beds, with each patient having their own room. Each MICU nurse was assigned to two patients. There was a central nursing station that kept track of the records, medications, and electronic recordings. Deidre was transferred from the day to the night shift. She found this shift more relaxing, with fewer phone calls and more autonomy. The job also paid more because of the hours. She didn't care; she had no one waiting at home. Most important, there were still plenty of interns and fellows to fool around with. It actually was too busy during the day. She tried to tease some of the more attractive residents by accidently rubbing up against them or having her nursing gown occasionally fly open and expose her breasts; but by and large, these things didn't work.

After a year on the night shift, Deidre's social life was not improving. She'd had plenty of forays with male aides and night nurses in vacated call rooms, but she made it clear that it was only sex and there was no future between them. So she came up with a better plan to get noticed.

If I made a heroic rescue of a patient, she thought to herself, *that might get me noticed.* So she cooked up a plan to inject one of her ICU patients with a toxic dose of epinephrine to induce a cardiac arrest. She would then be first on the scene to signal the arrest alert and to perform the initial emergency CPR, while waiting for the arrest team to arrive with the crash cart.

Deidre selected Mr. Patrick White as her victim. He was admitted for severe chronic obstructive pulmonary disease, the result of decades of smoking cigarettes. He was intubated and sedated as he lay in his hospital bed. Deidre went into the unit's pharmaceutical cabinet to retrieve vials of epinephrine. At the time, pharmaceuticals were kept in locked cabinets with paper documentation of utilization. This was before the installation of computerized medication management systems that require login and password entry to track orders and dispensements. Deidre was among the members of the ICU team who had keys to the medications cabinet.

Epinephrine is a class of drug termed "pressors." Epinephrine and norepinephrine are neurotransmitters and naturally occurring hormones that help regulate blood pressure. In times of extreme distress, epinephrine is used as a drug to constrict blood vessels from peripheral vessels, thereby increasing blood pressure to the central organs — the heart, brain, lungs, and liver — that are critical for life. It has been used to treat patients with cardiac arrest and anaphylaxis for many years. The standard dose for treatment of cardiac arrest is 10 milliliters of a 1:10,000 epinephrine concentration, totaling a 1 mg dose. At high concentrations, the effect of epinephrine is paradoxical: it induces cardiac arrest.

Deidre was taught all of these facts during nursing school. Now, she purposefully administered a high dose of epinephrine, 50 milliliters of a 1:10,000 concentration and waited in the ICU's break room for Mr. White to go into arrest. When the alarms went off just a few minutes later, she rushed to Mr. White's bedside acting surprised, and began chest compressions. The monitors on the nursing unit signaled an automatic response on the hospital's loudspeakers. "Cardiac arrest, MICU, bed three. Cardiac arrest, MICU, bed three." When the arrest team arrived, they found Deidre already hard at work on Mr. White trying to revive him. She stepped aside and allowed the team members to do their job. They tried defibrillation several times on Mr. White but failed to get any pulse or restart his breathing. After a half hour and much to the surprise of Deidre, the patient in bed three was dead. The whole objective of this exercise was to rescue Mr. White so that she would be the hero. Murder had not been her intent. But she was now at the point of no return. Mr. White was pronounced dead, and a sheet was drawn over his head. There was nobody in the morgue at 2:00 a.m., so they closed the door. Mr. White's body stayed in the unit until morning. The team thanked Deidre for her efforts. An autopsy was not conducted on Mr. White because he was elderly and had many medical problems. According to his wishes, his body was embalmed and he was buried alongside his wife who died two years earlier.

Although Deidre had just committed murder, she

couldn't believe the high she got from committing this atrocity. *This is better than any coke I've had in the past*, she thought to herself. It was ironic that the murder weapon was the same ingredient that was coursing through her veins and giving her the natural buzz. *I could do this again*, was her next thought.

There was no suspicion of foul play regarding the death of Mr. White. Deidre went about her business at the ICU without concern or remorse over his death. Several uneventful months went by. Then one weekend, she got a call from a resident she'd met a few weeks earlier in the hospital cafeteria one night. Dr. Ben Taylor was an obstetrics resident who had just delivered a baby in the hospital. It was a difficult breech delivery where the feet came out of the womb before the head. The mother was screaming in pain, but insisted that she wanted to deliver her child naturally so no epidural anesthesia was given. The ordeal wasn't over until well after midnight. Although he was tired, he was still wide awake because of the adrenaline rush of the baby's delivery. He knew Deidre was a night owl because of her hours and thought maybe she was available for a late dinner. Ben called the MICU and asked when Deidre was coming off her shift. The MICU was not full that night and Deidre only had one patient, Mrs. O'Toole, a 90-year old woman with end-stage congestive heart failure. She knew that if there were no patients, she could leave. So even though Mrs. O'Toole was still alive, she told Ben that she would be available in an hour. Deidre snuck into the pharmacy cabinet and took some vials of epinephrine. But this time, she injected a lethal dose into Mrs. O'Toole, who was quickly pronounced dead. With her out of the way, Diedre was able to sign out, and was available for her date with Ben. Nobody on the unit suspected any foul play. She now had a superiority complex over her patients. *I can control whether you live or die*, she said to herself. Her mental derangement was complete.

Deidre became fascinated with death and her control over people's lives. She reasoned that many of these poor unfortunate souls were on the verge of dying anyway and that she was simply helping them move on to their next appointment in eternity. Many of them did not appear to have family members who came around or cared about them. Of course she wouldn't really know this, since visitation hours were over before she started her night shift. Deidre was responsible for the death of countless patients in the MICU during the three years she worked there. Toward the end of Deidre's tenure there, her motivation for these actions changed to one of revenge for her lot in life. She was no longer involved in the resuscitation of patients. Only in their deaths.

*

Sarah Gellman worked in the General Hospital's Quality Control and Quality Assurance office. Part of her job was to review case records for unusual occurrences. Some of the things her group kept track of included success rates of surgical procedures, hospital-acquired infections, transplant rejection rates, medication errors, and in-hospital deaths. These statistics were disclosed to the state's medical board and became public information. Hospital ratings were based in part from these statistics. The General Hospital was listed in the top ten in the country in many of the medical fields. Sarah was proud of this fact and did her part to keep its reputation at a high level.

When she was reviewing the ICU records, one statistic seemed to jump off the page. The cardiac arrest rate from the MICU was much higher than in the other units. And it appeared to occur most often overnight, giving new meaning to the term "graveyard shift." *What was the common denominator*, Sarah asked herself. She first determined the medical service in charge of the case to see if there was something systematic. Sometimes it was a cardiology team, other times it was pulmonary and neurology teams. So that wasn't it. Then she looked at the nursing staff. There she found that in many of the deaths, a nurse Deidre Murphy was in charge. Deidre had a good employment record and was praised by many of the doctors on the unit. Sarah was careful not to incriminate a trusted employee without more evidence. So she contacted the charge nurse, Samantha Frasier, who was Sarah's friend and lunchtime running partner.

"What do you know about Deidre Murphy?" she asked Sam one day after lunch.

"Deidre works the third shift, so I only see her briefly in the morning, but by all accounts, she is an excellent ICU nurse. Why do you ask?"

Sarah told Sam that the MICU had a higher incidence of cardiac arrest than the national or regional average for facilities of comparable complexity, and that Deidre was the nurse on duty in a disproportionate number of those incidences.

"I can't prove this and I am not asking you to take any disciplinary action, but can you keep an eye on her?" Sam nodded and they parted.

Based on the reports, Sam suspected that Deidre was using epinephrine inappropriately on her ICU patients. Maybe she was using the wrong dosage on her patients when an order for epinephrine use was written? There were some vials missing from their accounting, but she figured it was just sloppy documentation. It was always chaotic during a cardiac arrest, and some of the paperwork may have been misplaced or overlooked. But now she realized that there likely was a more sinister reason for the missing vials. So Sam alerted the night nursing supervisor about Deidre and they secretly kept track of the number of dosages available. All of this suspicion was unbeknownst to Deidre.

Within six weeks, Deidre was planning her next victim. This time it was Mrs. Emily Rodriquez, a patient with terminal multiple sclerosis. After she died, Sam did an investigation and discovered empty vials of epinephrine in the ICU trash. There was no note in Mrs. Rodriquez's medical record that a resuscitation attempt had been made on her. Sam retrieved the vials and turned them over to the police for possible fingerprints, although she knew it was unlikely because all the nurses wore gloves when handling patients. So she could not absolutely prove that it was Deidre who was doing the killings. Nevertheless, Sam called Sarah the next day, who in turn contacted the hospital's lawyers and District Attorney Bobrick Kendall. Deidre was arrested on charges of murder and was removed from her job at the General Hospital. "Let's hope there are no more unexpected deaths on this unit now," Sarah said to Sam after the arrest.

In the investigation of the case, DA Kendall knew he only had circumstantial evidence against Deidre. Without an admission of guilt or more direct evidence that epinephrine injection was the cause of the cardiac arrest and subsequent death, the DA would have to let Deidre go free. I was called in to see if I could perform some postmortem testing that proved that epinephrine was administered to the patients who died under Deidre's care. The problem was that many of the bodies that she was alleged to have killed had been dead for months and, in some cases, years.

So I had to formulate a plan to prove or disprove the DA's case. An important complication was that epinephrine is a naturally occurring hormone that is released just prior to violent or so-called "agonal" deaths. Epinephrine release is part of a body's defense mechanism to extreme stress, sometimes called the "fight or flight" response. All of the MICU deaths occurred while the patients were unconscious, so there should not have been any natural hormone release. I also knew that "norepinephrine" was the precursor hormone to epinephrine. Norepinephrine was typically present at blood levels 5 times higher than epinephrine. These hormones metabolized to normetanephrine and metanephrine, respectively, and the ratio between these two metabolites was also 5 to 1. So an increased epinephrine or metanephrine concentrations along with a disproportionate ratio to norepinephrine or normetanephrine would suggest an epinephrine injection. I tested vitreous fluid from the eyes of victims instead of blood, as this was a better preserved specimen after death. As a "negative control," I got vitreous fluid from those who had natural deaths and compared the results against those of Mrs. Rodriquez. As a "positive control," I obtained vitreous fluids from patients who underwent epinephrine resuscitation just prior to death. Finally, since it is difficult to make definitive conclusions on a single poisoning case, DA

Kendall and I agreed to have the other bodies in question exhumed, and to perform vitreous samples testing on them. Permission was granted by the presiding judge and by each of the decedent's surviving family members; the graves were dug up. Intact eyes were delivered to the General Hospital's morgue, where I was able to extract vitreous fluid from three of the most recent victims. The fluids from some of the others had dried out so there was no sample to test. Not being a pathologist, I found it somewhat gruesome to extract fluid from those eyeballs, but I did it.

After several months of work, I was ready to present the findings to DA Kendall. Indeed, there were higher absolute concentrations of epinephrine and metanephrine metabolites in the suspicious deaths and in those who underwent epinephrine resuscitation than in the individuals who died of natural causes. But as I'd expected, there was a lot of variability in the results. The ratio between epinephrine and norepinephrine was considerably out of kilter. I concluded that this was evidence that a lethal injection took place. But I cautioned DA Kendall that these assays were not fully validated to be able to make this conclusion with one hundred percent certainty. I had been on the other side of the ledger many times – scientists who made scientific conclusions based on data that was not fully substantiated. I informed Kendall that no other epinephrine studies had yet been conducted on cadavers buried for months. An important issue was the stability of the compounds in question under these unusual conditions, although the calculation of ratio should correct for some instability assuming that epinephrine and norepinephrine degraded at the same rate.

157

Kendall agreed that if they presented this evidence in open court, the defendant's attorneys would likely contest the admissibility of the evidence. A ruling against the prosecution on this scientific point might be damaging to the credibility of the other more circumstantial evidence that was yet to be presented in this case.

DA Kendall decided not to use any of my data, and to proceed with the trial using the circumstantial evidence alone. The key to the case was the statistical aberration of the number of deaths that occurred while Deidre was on duty, so DA Kendall hired a statistician to provide expert testimony. Given that there were more deaths when Deidre was working than all of the other shifts combined, including her days off, vacations, and holidays, and just before she started her job at the General Hospital and after she left, the odds of the increased death rate being coincidental were one in over one hundred fifty million, according to the statistician's testimony. Then Dr. Ben Taylor testified that one of Deidre's patients coincidently died just minutes before his date with her, which suddenly made her available. This and other circumstantial evidence was sufficient in getting the jury to convict Deidre on three counts of murder. She was sentenced to five consecutive life sentences with no opportunity for parole. My work was not without influence. Based on my studies, the DA was totally convinced that Deidre was guilty. This prompted him and his team to work that much harder to deliver the proper justice. But in this case, the presentation of unproven data would have been worse than presenting no data at all.

*

After Deidre Murphy's conviction, her high school classmates said that they thought she was capable of these actions. Whether this was an accurate assessment of her character or some "after-the-fact" revision of history is unknown. Deidre was not the first to use epinephrine as a poison. Other nurses and healthcare workers have employed a similar approach, aided by unauthorized access to medications. Today, medications in hospitals are no longer available through locked cabinets. Computerized medication dispensers are prevalent across pharmacies, emergency departments, and intensive care units. Entry into these systems requires login and proper password documentation. All of these safeguards mean that the type of poisonings that were perpetrated by Deidre is less likely to occur today.

However, there are still ways to kill someone in a hospital. One non-drug related poison that remains a threat is potassium. An essential intracellular ion, intravenous potassium is commonly available for patients whose concentration of this electrolyte is deficient. However, an overdose injection of potassium chloride can immediately stop a heart. Lethal injections of potassium are used by some states as a means for executing prisoners on death row. As with epinephrine, murder with electrolytes is difficult to detect at autopsy. All cells have high concentrations of potassium that leak into post mortem blood due to the gradual breakdown of tissues after death.

The Vacationing Rapist

****

Rocky Alexander was the only child of a wealthy family. He was big for his age. The family owned a chain of hardware stores that littered the state. Even before he entered high school, Rocky spent his summers working in his father's central warehouse. His job was to load the inventory of goods that went out to the individual stores. This daily physical activity built up his muscles and kept him in good physical condition. Although he was the owner's kid, the other workers treated him like he was one of them. He liked being a part of a team. The guys would occasionally let Rocky drink beer with them after work.

At Stanleyville High School, Rocky was the football team's star linebacker. In his senior year, he led the team in tackles. They were undefeated going into the final game against their rival. A win would launch them into the state playoffs as the number one seed. It was a hard fought game. The opponent was driving for the go ahead touchdown with time running out and Rocky's team ahead by 5 points. The defensive coordinator called for a blitz. Rocky raced across the quarterback's blind side unabated, and was soon in the other team's backfield. When the quarterback was about to pass, Rocky knocked the ball loose. As it was falling onto the turf, Rocky's teammate recovered the ball. Stanleyville High secured the win. There was a wild celebration in the locker room, with the boys yelling and shouting. Bottles of soda were vigorously shaken, then opened and squirted over all of the players and coaches. The coach arranged a victory party for the team at a nearby farm. Rocky knew he would have a good time.

It seemed like the entire school was at the celebration. All the players from both the varsity and junior varsity football teams and the other sports teams were there. Even many of the players from the opposing team came. Of course there were plenty of girls, too, including the cheerleaders, the pep squad, and members of the marching band. The beer was flowing freely from the kegs. Guys were making out with the girls. Others were smoking pot in fields nearby. Everyone was dancing to the music blasting from the loudspeakers. Rocky was in the center of it all. This was his last year of school and he had a few games left. He made the key play today and knew that there were college scouts in attendance. While his family had plenty of money to pay for school, a football scholarship would heighten his on-campus notoriety.

*

Amy came to the party at the insistence of her best friend Tawny. Tawny's older brother and his girlfriend also went and drove them all there. Amy and Tawny, friends since kindergarten, were now 15-year-old freshmen. Tawny was outgoing and popular while Amy was quiet and reserved. Tawny convinced Amy that coming to this party would help her meet other kids and maybe get over her shyness. So she agreed and put on the prettiest outfit she owned. At the party, Amy did have fun. She saw a boy in her algebra class and the two of them got along well.

By one in the morning, the party was winding down. Many of the kids were passed out or heading home. Amy saw that it was late. When she went to find Tawny, she was surprised to find her kissing some boy she'd just met at the party.

Amy said to Tawny, "I'm tired, can we go home now? I told my mom I'd be back before one. Where's your brother?"

"He left with his girlfriend an hour ago," Tawny replied. "I want to stay. Can't you find your own ride home?" Amy was upset that she was being stranded and that Tawny was dumping her without a ride. She didn't want to call her mom to come and get her but she had no choice.

As she was pulling out her cellphone, a boy who overheard the conversation said, "I can take you home. I'm leaving now. Where do you live?" Amy recognized him as Rocky, the star of the football team. But she had never actually met him and wasn't sure this was a good idea.

"I'm going to call my mom, she doesn't mind coming to get me," Amy said, backing away slowly.

"Hey, don't you have an older sister named Sarah?" Rocky asked. He was thinking about how hot Sarah was; she had a reputation for being easy.

"Yeah. She's at State College now," Amy said, feeling a bit more comfortable since Rocky knew her sister.

"So are you coming? The bus is leaving," he said. Rocky had a kind face and everybody knew him. So she said, sure. He drove a Range Rover that was parked nearby. They got in and Amy told him where she lived. Rocky, a little drunk, pulled out and headed back to town. After a few minutes, he pulled off to the side of the road to a deserted spot, turned off the engine, and unbuckled his seatbelt.

"Did you have a good time there, baby?"

Amy nervously replied, "Yes I did. But, I'm really tired now, so can we go?"

"But don't you want some of this first?" he asked, pointing to just below his waist.

"No, what do you think you are doing? Stop, I just want to go home!" Undeterred, Rocky reached over, unbuckled her seatbelt and got on top of her. "Not until we're done," he shouted. Amy started screaming, begging him to get off of her. Rocky struck her in the face with his hand and said, "Shut up, bitch. You know you want this." Not wanting to be harmed any more, Amy stopped resisting and started to cry. Rocky reclined her seat, ripped off her clothes, and violently raped her. Being a virgin, she began to bleed, with blood running down her leg. When he was finished, he put his pants back on, got back into the driver's seat and drove her home. Amy was quietly sobbing in the seat next to him.

When she got out, he gave her a warning, saying sternly, "Don't you tell anyone about this or the next time it'll be worse." Amy got out, ran into her house and went straight to her room. Her parents heard her come home but were in bed almost asleep. She took off her torn dress, got into the shower and with the water running, sat on the floor of the shower crying.

The next morning, she was afraid to say anything to her parents, remembering Rocky's threat. Tawny came over to tell Amy about her night. But Tawny noticed that Amy was upset and asked her what happened. Amy broke down and told Tawny everything.

"He raped me in his car. My life is ruined." Tawny hugged her but Amy pushed her away. "It's your fault entirely. I knew I shouldn't have gone," she cried.

"You have to tell, Tawny said. "We'll get that bastard. A lot of people saw him leave with you. We need to call the cops. Right now!" After much reluctance, Amy told her parents and they immediately called the police. Amy's parents then took her to the emergency department of a local hospital where she was examined in a private room with a female nurse and doctor. Her vaginal area was swabbed. The swab was sealed, signed, and sent to the police laboratory for evidence of semen. Amy was embarrassed about doing all of this. Her parents said it was necessary. The lab tested the swab for the presence of acid phosphatase, an enzyme found in male ejaculate. The result was positive, confirming that intercourse occurred, and was reported to the police.

Rocky was at home when the Stanleyville police arrived. He was arrested for rape. Rocky denied the charge and said that Amy had consented. His family put up the $100,000 bond. News got out around school. The star football player was accused of rape. An arraignment was scheduled for two weeks later. Amy would not return to the school where she and Rocky were attending. She returned only on the day of the arraignment. She dreaded having to face her rapist but her father said it was necessary. The courtroom opened, the judge, DA, and defense attorneys were present. But there was no sign of Rocky. His family didn't know where he was or why he wasn't there. A warrant was issued to find and detain Rocky for trial. But he was gone.

For twelve years, Rocky went missing. Rocky's family denied knowledge of his whereabouts. The town gradually forgot about this case and people moved on with their lives. Everyone except Gus Holmes, who was Stanleyville's detective in charge of investigating assaults. Gus tried everything to locate Rocky's whereabouts. None of his friends knew where he'd gone.

After years of no leads, Gus finally got a lucky break. One of his colleagues at the police station was traveling in Europe on vacation and saw a movie about a ski instructor working in a resort in the French Alps. On the end credits, one of the film's extras was listed as Rocky Alexander. He got a copy of the movie, and showed it to Gus when he returned. "That's him," Gus said after studying the film frame by frame. Rocky was only in one scene. "Older and sporting a mustache. I can't believe he was so arrogant as to appear in this film and to use his real name in the film credits," Gus said.

With support from his family, Rocky spent the last decade living in northern France. He held odd jobs as a ski instructor, bartender, and waiter. He never changed his name but he did make a new life for himself. He told his family that he was innocent of rape. That she came on to him and the sex was consensual. But he and his family didn't think he could get a fair trial so he fled. Interpol was contacted and Rocky was extradited back to the U.S. to stand trial.

Rocky's family hired the best lawyer that money could buy. Carrolton Smyth III assisted on the OJ Simpson defense team as a junior lawyer. He was the one who reviewed the blood spot data at the scene of Nicole Simpson's death and concluded that since trace amounts of EDTA — a common anticoagulant in blood collection tubes — was present, the blood on OJ's clothing was previously collected and planted by the Los Angeles police. Now a full partner in his law firm, he told the Alexander family that he could get Rocky acquitted.

Rocky's Range Rover was impounded by the police immediately after the rape accusation. There was a single blood spot on the carpet. Investigators removed that part of the rug and sent it to the crime laboratory, where it was tested for the owner's identity. Just after the rape, Amy underwent a physical examination. Traces of Rocky's semen were recovered from her body and clothes. Amy knew that the blood in the car was hers. The Stanleyville District Attorney, Thomas Washington, told her that a DNA match would establish where the rape occurred. So she willingly gave a fresh blood sample, hoping this would convict him. She didn't think a jury would believe Rocky's story that she enticed him to have sex with her. As this was her first time, why would she give in to someone she hadn't even met before?

The defense requested that the dried blood spots be tested for the presence of drugs. They announced their findings to DA Washington just before the trial started. A hearing in front of the judge was scheduled to determine the admissibility of the evidence according to the Frye criteria: evidence must have scientific credibility before it can be presented to a jury. A prominent toxicologist, Dr. Harold McMaster, was hired by the defense to explain the lab results.

Smyth opened the testimony. "Dr. McMaster, the DNA evidence has established that these blood spots belong to Amy. We are not disputing that Rocco and Amy had sex in the vehicle on the night in question. What else did the toxicology lab find in these blood spots?"

McMaster replied, "The lab found traces of tetrahydrocannabinol in her blood. We believe she was smoking marijuana at the party and was high at the time of intercourse." Smyth concluded, "This is evidence of reckless behavior and shows that the sex was not rape."

Amy was shocked to hear this accusation against her. She never smoked pot back then or at any other time since. "I can't believe this is happening to me," she said to her attorney. "They're twisting it to say it's my fault."

Thomas Washington contacted me to review the defense's toxicology data and testify as to the validity of these conclusions. "This immunoassay is a screening test that requires confirmation testing by mass spectrometry."

"There was insufficient blood left to do the confirmation test," McMaster said.

"Without this second test, it is my opinion this data has no scientific validity. The immunoassay test has never been used before on dried blood spots recovered from a carpet, especially blood that is 12 years old," I said to the judge.

DA Washington concluded, "Since the confirmatory mass spectrometry test was not conducted, these results cannot be entered into evidence, as it would be prejudicial."

Unfortunately, the judge did not agree with the DA and allowed the evidence to be heard. The trial proceeded. The blood spot evidence put sufficient doubt into four of the 12 juror's minds, resulting in a hung jury. No verdict. Back to square one for the DA. The DA was committed to retrying — and convicting — Rocky for rape.

Realizing that the carpet toxicology data was slim, Smyth wanted to find a new angle for the new trial. Examining the evidence list, he noted that the crime lab had Amy's underwear. Since the panties contained her blood stains, he ordered new toxicology tests. This time, he directed the new lab to only use mass spectrometry, the confirmatory procedure. McMaster presented the new toxicology test results and during this trial the conclusion was that Amy had taken heroin that night! Amy couldn't believe how her reputation was increasingly being assassinated. First weed and now heroin? She told the DA, "I wasn't on any drugs that night or any night. Who's the victim here?"

At that point she looked straight into my eyes. Through the tears and without speaking, her eyes were saying *Help me. Please help me.* From that point forward, I was in. I was going to do my best to get that bastard. This is not the proper attitude for an impartial expert witness and I wasn't going to twist facts. But nevertheless, I was all in.

I was again asked to review and possibly refute the data. In court, I stated, "While mass spectrometry was used in testing these blood spots, the lab did not follow forensic procedures. Heroin cannot be detected in blood, as it breaks down too quickly. What was allegedly found, morphine, was below the lab's stated limit of detection. If morphine was present, and I am not saying it was, it could have simply been from codeine use, since morphine is the breakdown product.

Smyth jumped in, saying, "Why would a healthy 15-year-old girl be on morphine? So what if it's not heroin, she was still abusing drugs."

I countered, "I said codeine. This is a common medication available through prescription. It is present in a variety of products that teenagers may use for a common cold or menstrual cramps. None of this matters, though, because the analysis was flawed."

The judge then said, "Continue with your testimony, doctor. What did you find?"

"The defendant's hired lab found a peak in the data that they suggested was morphine. Looking at the data, I saw that the peak appeared buried among the background noise and that a digital smoothing technique was used to make it appear more like a real peak." I then pulled out one of my own charts. "In this graph, a similar peak is present using the same analytical conditions and smoothing algorithm. However, in this case, this chart is a sample of pure distilled water. In order to confirm the presence of a drug, multiple fragment ions must be present. That technique was not used on Amy's blood." I then went on to say, "We have subsequently learned that this test was conducted in a private garage laboratory in Houston, Texas. We sent an investigator there. Here is a picture of the house. This lab has no certification or credibility. It's basically a lab for hire." I am not normally this animated when testifying when testifying and usually don't take sides. But I knew this creep was guilty and didn't want him to be exonerated without a fight. It was getting personal. Besides, I felt like they deserved it for what they were doing to Amy.

Smyth jumped up and shouted, "I object to the last

statement. The witness is adding his personal opinions."

The judge ruled, "Sustained. The jury will disregard the last statement by the witness."

Shortly after my testimony, both sides rested their case and the jury was sequestered for their verdict. After two days, word got out that a decision had been reached and was soon to be announced. I normally don't get personally involved in cases nor do I attend the announcement of the verdict. But in this case, several of my colleagues in the toxicology field purposely misrepresented toxicology data. So as the jury was about to reassemble, I was there and never felt more nervous. I hoped that my arguments were sufficiently convincing. I could feel my heart pounding. The members of the jury returned in single file and took their seats, eyes cast downward. No eye contact was made between any member of the jury and Rocky.

Smyth said to himself, *this is never a good sign.*

Once seated, the judge asked, "Mr. Foreman has the jury reached a verdict?"

"We have your honor. In the matter of rape, we rule the defendant," he paused slightly and then continued, "is guilty as charged." Rocky slumped into his seat. Having been shown that Amy was not on any drug, the jury was convinced that the sex occurred against her will.

The judge then said, "The court thanks the jury for your work in this case. The defendant will be held for sentencing. Given his history, bail is denied." Amy hugged DA Washington and they walked out of the courtroom.

"But, but, I didn't rape that girl," Rocky said repeatedly, as he was escorted out of the courtroom. "She wanted it."

Rocky Alexander was sentenced to 20 years. He was up for parole after eight. When he answered the parole panel's questions, it was clear that Rocky still believed in his innocence. "The sex was consensual." Amy was present at the proceedings but wasn't asked to testify. Parole was denied and Rocky served another six years before he was finally released. He was now 44 years old. His last football game was 26 years earlier. The DA considered arresting his parents on an obstruction of justice charge, suspecting that they must have supported Rocky during his years in France. But there was insufficient evidence to pursue the case, and it was never filed. Amy married and had two children. She never forgave Rocky for that night. When her kids are old enough, Amy will tell them about what happened to her.

*

In the time between Rocky Alexander's two rape trials, the standard for admissibility of scientific evidence shifted from the "Frye Test" to the "Daubert Standard." In the first trial, the judge ruled that the blood stain on the carpet was not admissible because the methodology used in the testing was not generally accepted by the scientific community. The judge in the second trial was held to the Daubert Standard, whereby the conclusion of an expert witness was qualified if it was a product of sound scientific methodology. Since mass spectrometry is accepted for forensic testing, the toxicology data in Amy's case was allowed in the second trial..

This case regarding Amy's rape was ultimately proven to not be drug-related. We did not find any credible evidence that Amy took any drugs prior to the assault, either purposefully or unwillingly. However, drug-induced date rape has become an issue for young adults. There are a number of drugs and chemicals that are used on unsuspecting victims for the purpose of a sexual assault. These drugs produce a sedative and hypnotic effect so that the victims become delirious and may be unaware of or defenseless to a rape. Because victims often are amnesic to the assault, perpetrators frequently escape identification and prosecution. In addition to alcohol, which has been used for date rape for centuries, contemporary "date rape" drugs include Rohypnol, ketamine, and gamma hydroxybutyrate (GHB). These are spiked into drinks of potential victims. Rohypnol is a sedative that is no longer approved for use in the U.S., but is available in other countries. In response to the use of Rohypnol as a date rape drug, the manufacturer has added a dye that produces a blue color when added to a clear drink, which has helped reduce the incidence of date rape. Ketamine, a tranquilizer used by veterinarians, is abused more in Southeast and East Asian countries than in the U.S. GHB, which was removed from the FDA-approved drug list in 1990, is a date rape drug that is also frequently abused by body builders as it induces the release of growth hormone.

Mushroom Rage

****

Sam Lewis grew up in the tough south side of Chicago. He didn't know his father, and his mother worked two jobs to keep him housed and fed. His mother tried to keep Sam out of trouble but she wasn't home a lot. When she got laid off, she became a prostitute. Sam was constantly challenged while in school and in his neighborhood. He learned to fight in order to defend himself. He dropped out of school at the age of 15. He started stealing from neighborhood stores. He got caught by the police and was sent to juvenile detention. There, he began to lift weights and hung out with other boys who had similar interests. Since Sam seemed to like confrontations, one of the counselors there told Sam about a boxing club in town. The counselor hoped that this could be a constructive outlet for his aggression. When he was released, he went to Benz Gym to check it out. Sebby Williams was the manager of the gym. Sebby had grown up in the same neighborhood 10 years earlier, and could relate to Sam. The counselor at the detention center told Sebby that Sam might be stopping by. When he arrived, the two of them hit it off immediately. Sam became a regular member of the fighting club. He didn't have any money so Sebby offered him a part time job cleaning the locker rooms.

Over the next several years, Sam became very proficient

at boxing. When Sam turned 18, Sebby arranged some bouts with fighters at other gyms as a middleweight. Sam won all of these fights, knocking out his opponent a fair number of times. Sebby sensed that Sam could become a successful professional fighter. He devoted more and more time towards training Sam and less time as the manager of the gym. Others within the boxing community began to take note. Sam's personality also transitioned from the local tough guy to someone who had a future. Sebby and his girlfriend Darlene asked Sam to move in with them as they had a spare room in their apartment. From then on, the three of them became inseparable. Darlene started to manage Sam's diet. Sebby sought out sponsors for Sam's fighting career. He was successful in getting some money from a local hardware store. A few years later, Sebby was able to quit his job at the Benz Gym and devote all of his time towards Sam's boxing future.

Sebby scheduled a big fight on Valentine's Day between Sam and another up and coming fighter from Detroit. His opponent was older and a more experienced boxer than Sam. Nevertheless, he was no match for Sam who was quicker and stronger. During the third round, Sam struck his opponent hard on the mouth and the left cheek. His mouth was bleeding profusely. The referee stopped the fight briefly in order for his team to attend to his wounds. When the fight resumed, Sam struck him again causing him to fall. At that point, Sam scored a technical knockout of his opponent. Members of the Benz Gym attending the fight were cheering for his success. Sebby felt that Sam's career was launched that night with the fight.

Later, Darlene hosted a party at their apartment to

celebrate Sam's success. Several members of the local boxing establishment were present. There was loud music and plenty of alcohol, marijuana, and cocaine. By three o'clock in the morning, all of their guests left. Darlene was tired and went to her room. Sam was still energized from his victory and from the methamphetamine he had been taking that evening. He was also drinking a special tea from a hallucinogenic mushroom that Sam got from a friend. Darlene brewed them from the pieces. Shortly thereafter, Sam became delirious and highly agitated

He shouted out at Sebby and pointed his index finger directly at him. "You are the devil! You are the devil!" Sebby was half asleep on the couch and paid no attention to Sam. Sam's eyes were wide open and glazed. He appeared to look past Sebby as he repeated his ramblings.

"Relax and have another drink" Sebby said as he stood up and looked up at Sam. Sam went into the kitchen and Sebby figured he was going to the refrigerator for a cold beer. Instead, Sam came back with a large kitchen knife.

Sebby was startled. "What are you doing with that?" he asked.

"Satan! Satan! You must be terminated!" With that, he lunged at Sebby and stabbed his manager in the chest. Sebby fell back into the couch, blood pouring out of his abdomen. Sam stabbed Sebby seventeen more times in the chest. By then Sebby was long gone. Still delirious, Sam excised Sebby's heart with the knife and shouted "You're the devil! Die, die, die!" He then threw the bloodied heart into the lit fireplace of their apartment. Sam then opened Sebby's mouth and cut out his tongue from the base. This was thrown into the fire too.

Darlene heard the commotion in the living room, got up from the bed and quietly cracked open the bedroom door. She was horrified to see what Sam did. She had never seen him or anybody else act like that before. She feared that she would be Sam's next victim. She locked her bedroom door ran, into her closet and hid behind some hung clothes hoping that Sam would not come after her. She could not get out the window because they were in a third floor apartment and the fire escape was on the other side of the apartment. But Sam didn't enter the bedroom. After an hour of silence, Darlene was brave enough to come out of the bedroom and saw that Sam was passed out in the living room. She grabbed her cell phone and ran out of the apartment to call 9-1-1. The police arrived within minutes, woke up Sam and took him into custody. The chief medical examiner was called to the scene. He and the police detectives meticulously took photographs of the scene and cataloged all of the evidence. Sebby's body was taken to the morgue. Darlene was asked to recount what happened that night. She was still visibly shaken but described what she saw and heard.

*

About sixteen months after the incident, I got the call from the district attorney, Harrison Belmont, who explained the case to me. I heard about it from newspaper reports. They wanted a toxicology laboratory to examine the evidence. "The decedent's girlfriend testified that the defendant was drinking a tea that she made. She also said that Sam was taking methamphetamine. The medical examiner has already verified the presence of methamphetamine and amphetamine from Sam's blood and urine taken the night that he was arrested. We need to know what is in the mushrooms."

"There are a number of mushrooms that contain hallucinogenic chemicals. What evidence do you have?"

"We have some tea leaves that were confiscated at the crime scene. There are some tall glasses that Darlene used to serve the tea. We also have vomitus from the carpet" Belmont explained.

"Why is it important that we prove he was drinking hallucinogenic mushrooms?" I asked. "He is obviously guilty."

"A public defender and his aide were assigned to Sam Lewis' case. They are going to plead temporary insanity, despite the fact that he has no history of mental illness. If we can prove that he willingly consumed a hallucinogenic mushroom, he would be culpable for his actions that night and we would charge him with murder. We are also going to argue that he was in a "roid rage" due to the excessive methamphetamine concentrations in his blood. If we can also show that he was also delirious due to the mushrooms, it would explain how he mistook Sebby for Satan. The medical examiner was unable to find any hallucinogenic chemicals in either Sam's or Sebby's blood. They did not test the exhibits recovered from the crime scene because our crime lab does not have the analytical capability of finding these chemicals. What do you think we can look for?"

"The most common psychedelic mushrooms are the psilocybins. Their hallucinogenic properties have been known and used by native Mexicans for centuries" I told Belmont.

"Can you examine dried blood spots from the victim for the presence of psilocybin?" the DA asked me. "We have sections from the couch and cushions that are soaked with Sebby

Williams' blood." Belmont then removed photographs taken at the scene of the crime to show me.

As a laboratory scientist, my technologists work with tubes of blood every day. However, seeing blood spots and tissue fragments as part of a gruesome crime scene caused me to wince a little. I gathered myself and told the DA, "Psilocybin is very unstable and quickly metabolizes to psilocin. How was the evidence stored?"

"Locked in evidence bags and stored in the evidence room at room temperature" Belmont responded.

I was not surprised by the answer. Ideally, biological samples should be stored frozen to minimize degradation. The police do not have refrigerators or freezers to keep evidence. "We'll do the best we can" I responded.

Mass spectrometry is a very powerful technique that can detect the smallest quantities of chemicals. We have used this technique for many years to measure hormone levels from dried blood spots of newborn infants. Every state in the U.S. has a newborn screening program. Physicians put a few drops of blood onto a card and mail them to the laboratory after the spots have dried. Through these tests, diseases such as phenylketonuria and congenital adrenal hyperplasia are detected within the first few days of life. Infants with these diseases are prescribed special diets that prevent complications. We have tested dried blood spots that have been stored at room temperature for many years without a problem, I thought to myself. But I was not sure this has ever been done for mushroom testing on a murder case.

I put one of my best analysts, Colby Maine, to the problem. We had standards and have measured psilocybin in mushrooms before. We had no problem finding psilocybin in the tea leaves and within the dried residues of the glasses that Sam and Sebby drank that night. However, we were not able to find any psilocybin or psilocin in any of the dried blood spots or vomitus. I told Belmont that it was very possible that these chemicals had degraded during the 16 months of storage in the police's evidence room. The other evidence suggested that at least Sam drank this tea.

Darlene testified during the trial that she gave both men the mushroom-laced tea just prior to her going to bed. Neither of them was acting strangely at the time. However, within 25 minutes, Sam's behavior changed dramatically. During his arrest, Sam told the police that he saw angels in the room. Users of psilocybin have described increased visual perception and strange light phenomena. When he looked over at Sebby, he saw no halos and mistook him as the devil. He became fearful. A voice told him he had to remove the demon. A medical toxicologist and mycologist testified that this account was consistent with acute psilocybin ingestion. The defense team confirmed our data for the presence of psilocybin in the leaves and drinking glasses collaborating Darlene's testimony. They did not hire their own toxicologist and did not challenge our findings. The DA offered Sam's defense team a guilty plea with life imprisonment without possibility of parole in lieu of a death sentence. Sam and his lawyers accepted the deal. I was grateful that I was not asked to appear on the stand to defend our data. I did not want to be in the same room as someone who had committed such a heinous act.

*

Psilocybin as a toxin is found in about 180 different species of mushrooms. There are some groups in North, Central and South America that regularly consume these mushrooms as part of religious ceremonies. This practice dates back to the era of the Mayans where statuettes have been found carved into the shape of these mushrooms. Natives believe that their use connects themselves with the divine in a mystical and transcendental manner.

Recreational use as a hallucinogen is a more recent practice. In 2006, the National Institute on Drug Abuse sponsored a double blind clinical trial on the physiologic and psychological effects of psilocybin onto 36 psilocybin-naïve adults. These investigators showed that most participants experienced increased well-being and life satisfaction. These effects lasted well beyond the initial period of intoxication. Other studies have demonstrated antidepressant effects of psilocybin among patients with obsessive-compulsive disorders and clinical depression. However, in the NIDA-sponsored trial, a few subjects experienced paranoia while on the drug.

This case demonstrated the dangers of mixing compounds that have different pharmacologic effects, i.e., a hallucinogen and a stimulant. There may have been synergistic effects that altered Sam's cognitive reasoning and vision, causing him to commit these acts. While this crime was not premeditated, the fighter was necessarily culpable for his actions.

Slide Toxin

Harrison Wang grew up in Palo Alto and was the son of Stanford professors. His father was a professor of immunology and his mom, a gastroenterologist at Stanford Hospital. His parents were from Taiwan and came to the U.S. when Harrison was a small child. Harrison excelled in the sciences while attending Gunn High School. When it came to college, everyone naturally assumed he would enroll at Stanford. When he applied, he did not disclose to the admissions committee that both his parents were professors there. He wanted to get in on his own merit. He got an offer from them, but to everyone's surprise, he turned down Stanford and attended the University of California at Berkeley.

"Cal" was the main athletic rival to Stanford when it came to sports. But Harrison wasn't interested in the sports teams and concentrated on his studies. Harrison majored in biomedical engineering. He spent his summers working for a cardiologist at UC San Francisco, and had an idea for a new sensor that was inserted into the body and provided important metabolic information for patients who have diabetes.

After college, Harrison debated about going to medical school or starting his own company. He had just gotten married to Kasey, his high school sweetheart from Gunn High School who also attended UC Berkeley. Rather than facing a decade of debt, he went the entrepreneur route. With the help of a cardiologist, he and a fellow Cal student founded "Fat Help Diagnostics, LLC." Within a year, they built a prototype device. It was tested on a rat model where diabetes was induced by the streptozotocin, a naturally occurring chemical that is toxic to the pancreas. Medical devices require a large investment of funds. Harrison got connected with the group, Y Combinator, who taught entrepreneurs how to get funding for startup companies like his. They were interested in Harrison because they knew that metabolic syndrome was increasing in incidence among baby boomers, including themselves. With the preliminary data generated from the prototype instrument, Y- Combinator assisted in getting Fat Help $10 million from other investors, making their company solvent for the next 5 years.

When they started human trials, most of Fat Help's early diagnostic devices failed due to mild allergic reactions from the materials used. Harrison's father suggested an immunologically neutral material, which helped them come up with a more promising prototype for humans. Satisfied with the human allergy data, they were ready to start a pilot human study. These trials are very complex and expensive. Fat Help needed a new round of funding. Harrison learned of a company in China who was willing to back them for a pilot study. Harrison traveled to Shanghai in the summer of 2013 to discuss possible financial support.

Harrison arrived in China and spent the afternoon in the Bund shopping for something for Kasey. He got her a large pink freshwater pearl necklace. Shopping also took his mind off the presentation he was to give the next day to a room full of corporate leaders. He was 25 but he still looked like a kid. The next day, he met with the CEO and CFO of the largest distributor of medical devices in China. Harrison's ability to speak Mandarin was a major advantage. *All those weekends of Chinese language lessons when he was a kid finally paid off,* he thought to himself. The Chinese executives loved Harrison's proposal and they drew up papers to support the preliminary study. There was a big dinner party that night in his honor. Every few minutes, another executive from the company came to him for a toast of sake wine. Harrison never drank so much but he couldn't be rude to his new partners. The next day, he was anxious to return to the Bay Area to be with Kasey and to break the good news to his colleagues.

Harrison flew to China in business class, but he changed his flight plan to leave Shanghai a day early, so only a coach class ticket was available. He agreed to sit on the exit row, on the left side of the plane, right behind the main cabin door in the middle seat. Seated next to him on the window seat, was Kirk, a 30-year old writer who was taking his first international flight. Harrison could see that Kirk was very nervous about this flight. Kirk read and memorized all of the safety precautions. He asked several questions of the flight attendants before and after making their usual safety announcements.

"How do I know the oxygen mask will come down when needed?" he asked.

"Don't worry, every plane is tested for this on a regular basis" the flight attendant said.

"What do you mean when the Captain says arm doors and cross check?"

The flight attendant said patiently, "It enables the automatic deployment of the evacuation chute. In the case of an emergency, the slide will automatically inflate when the plane door is opened."

Harrison did his best to calm Kirk down. Once they were airborne, Harrison asked Kirk "Why don't you have a beer? I'm buying."

But even after the brew, Kirk kept fidgeting. He kept Harrison awake during this first flight segment. *Maybe he'll get off in Seoul, our first stop,* Harrison thought to himself. No such luck, when they landed, it was clear that Harrison and Kirk would be accompanying each other all the way to San Francisco.

The second leg of the flight was not as bad as Harrison thought. Once the plane departed, Kirk fell asleep and was calm during most of the trip. When it was time to land at SFO, they were instructed to turn off electronics, move the seat to the upright position, tighten seat belts, and return trays to the upright position. The plane was about to land. Kirk was looking out the window and saw the plane's approach towards the runway.

"Doesn't it look like we're too low?" We're still over water and I don't see the runway!" he said to Harrison. Harrison ignored him; all he could think of was Kasey waiting for him at the airport. But the plane was flying too low. Just before touching down, the engines roared suddenly. The pilot was trying to abort the landing. The plane suddenly tipped upwards but it was too late. The back of the plane crashed into the rocks just ahead of the runway. Then it rocked from side to side and

186

then the front of the plane came crashing down. There was an explosion as the back of the airplane disappeared, and there was a loud screeching noise of metal hitting the concrete runway. Harrison and the other passengers lunged forward against their seat belt. Luggage fell out of the overhead bins. Oxygen masks were automatically released. After a few seconds, the plane came to an abrupt halt. Harrison noticed that blood was coming out of his ears from the trauma.

The pilot, unaware of the extent of the damage, told everyone to remain calm and in their seats. But Kirk would not listen. He jumped out of his seat and began to unlock the cabin door to the outside. The flight attendants got up and demanded that he return to his seat.

"The plane is going is explode soon, we must get out!" cried Kirk.

Then there was a struggle between Kirk and a male flight attendant. Harrison got up and tried to restrain Kirk. But it was no good. Kirk managed to open the door to a halfway position. When the door was opened, the chute began to inflate. Instead of swinging the door completely open, Kirk quickly closed the door, and the evacuation chute deployed inside the plane. Kirk was off to the side when it opened. Harrison, on the other hand, was directly behind the slide and was knocked onto the ground by its sudden inflation. He hit his head on the floor of the plane and was unconscious. Right around that time, the pilot announced that everyone was to immediately evacuate the plane. Flames erupted near the back of the plane, which had a gaping hole. Several of the passengers fell onto the tarmac, still belted to their seats. Kirk grabbed his carry on bag and ran towards the midsection of the plane and was able to escape. At first, no one noticed that Harrison was trapped under the inflated slide. Within 90 seconds, most of the passengers escaped the plane. One of the last flight attendants saw a leg peeking out from the failed chute. *Someone is trapped underneath! she thought.* The attendant grabbed a knife from the galley and cut into the chute to deflate it. She and one of the pilots carried Harrison off the plane.

*

The accident occurred on a Saturday morning. I was playing golf with my friends as I normally do on weekends. I got the call when I was putting on the 17th green. *Who could this be?* It was the lab. There had been a plane crash at San Francisco Airport. Casualties will be coming to my hospital. My staff was trained for mass casualties, but it was mostly in the context of an earthquake or other natural disasters.

"Do we have enough staff to handle this?" was my first reaction.

"Yes" said Roxy, who was the chemistry lab supervisor who came in that day to catch up with her work. *Thank god I have someone from my senior management staff there,* I thought. *She will be able to bring in extra human resources if they are needed."*

"There are not very many who have serious injuries" she said to me over the phone. She continued, "The blood bank will be busy, but we will probably only get test requests for blood gases and electrolytes. Bray, our facilities manager, is coming in and will prepare a cart of extra lab supplies like phlebotomy tubes, and will be dropping them off at the ED for their immediate use."

*

Harrison was taken to the General Hospital in serious condition in one of the first ambulances. He suffered head trauma and other physical injuries during the fall. There was also a question of smoke inhalation as he was one of the last persons to be evacuated. By then the interior of the plane filled with smoke. Over the course of the next few days, Harrison's medical condition worsened. He was profoundly hypotensive and was treated with pressors. He suffered a head injury as the result of his fall. His eardrums were ruptured. His intracranial pressure was very high requiring a surgical shunt to relieve the pressure. Drugs were given to reduce his metabolic demands. The next day, he developed rhabdomyolysis, extensive skeletal muscle injury as the result of his trauma. This caused the release of skeletal muscle enzymes and proteins such as myoglobin, which led to obstruction of his kidney tubules resulting in failure of this organ. He was treated with dialysis used to temporarily replace his normal renal function. Kasey and Harrison's parents took turns being at bedside throughout the time he was at the General. After two days, he unexpectedly developed a significant metabolic acidosis due to the accumulation of lactic acid. Because of the delayed onset of his acidosis, the poison control center was contacted to determine if there were acids or toxins that could explain his latest symptoms.

I got a call from Terrance Norris, head of the Northern California Poison Center. He asked me "What do you know about sodium azide exposure?"

"Sodium azide is a bactericide widely used as a preservative in our chemical reagents" I responded. "It is highly explosive and we have to take precautions in the lab when using it and disposing it. Why do you ask?"

"We have some very sick passengers from the weekend's plane crash. One of them may have been exposed."

Azide is used to automatically inflate automobile airbags after a traffic accident. There are only a few grams in the bag of a car. This chemical is also used to inflate airplane evacuation chutes. These slides require kilogram quantities of azide because of the larger volume of gas needed for inflation.

"One of our patients was trapped beneath the air bag chute that opened inside the plane" Terrance continued. "We are thinking that when the bag was opened and deflated, our patient may have inhaled some of the unreacted azide remaining in the bag" Terrance explained. "We'd like for you to test his blood for azide."

"I am familiar with a fatality involving sodium azide reported in the literature. Azide can interrupt energy production leading to hypotension and a cardiac arrest." I responded. "We don't have a laboratory test for this right now, but I will see if we can put something together real quick."

"Thanks. Poisoning by azide in this case is a long shot, but we don't have anything else to go on" Terrance concluded.

I received this call in the late morning, one hour before a schedule appointment with Donna Late, a representative of the company who makes our analytical instrumentation. In reviewing the literature for methods, I noticed that we were missing a critical reagent needed for us to do the test. To order this chemical would have delayed testing for at least 1-2 days. So I asked Donna if they had the reagent back in their labs that I could borrow in an emergency. They told me they knew of a research lab nearby who might have this chemical. I contacted the lab director who found it on their shelves. Shortly after the original request by the poison center was received, Jen from my staff developed a working assay for azide and hydrazoic acid, formed when azide contacts water. The admission samples from Harrison and other crash victims seen at the General Hospital were examined. We knew approximately what the toxic concentration would be in blood from the literature reports. A standard was prepared from a bottle of sodium azide that we had in the lab. After careful examination, all of the blood samples including those of Harrison had absolutely no trace of sodium azide or hydrazoic acid. I was somewhat relieved to know that this was not the cause of Harrison's medical problems, imagining that this could spurn a series of lawsuits from car crash victims. After searching for a number of other chemicals and substances, we concluded that there were no toxic exposures during the plane crash that were responsible for Harrison's clinical problems.

Harrison died four days after admission due to his injuries. He never regained consciousness. The news media were notified and a press conference was called. The lead critical care physician attending to Harrison's care broke the news. Within two hours, the medical examiner sent a courier and an aide who came into my laboratory requesting all left over blood samples from the decedent for their postmortem investigation.

"These samples will be important to The National Transportation Safety Board's investigation of the accident" said the representative from the ME's office.

"Care for our current patients takes priority over your retrospective postmortem" I told them. "What we find in Mr.

Harrison's blood may be useful for those who are still alive and in our ICU. Some of them have the same medical problems. We will turn over these blood samples once we have completed our analysis." Satisfied with that answer, they left my office. They came back a few weeks later and I gave them the remaining samples.

Kacey found the pink pearl necklace among Harrison's luggage when they were returned to her by NTSB and knew that Harrison was thinking of her when the plane went down. She fell to her knees and cried quietly in her bedroom. She wore the necklace at his funeral and it was a sharp contrast to the black outfit she was wearing. Harrison's remains were laid to rest about 100 yards from Steve Jobs, who was buried in the same cemetery two years earlier. The two entrepreneurs were very much alike. But one fulfilled his destiny while the other had his cut short before it got started.

*

Airbags, technically known as air cushion restraint systems were invented in 1951 and were originally inflated by compressed air. It was not until 1967 that sodium azide was used as the means for inflation. Airbags appeared in consumer vehicles in the early 1970s on a limited basis and as an option. Porsche was the first car manufacturer to make the airbag standard equipment in 1987. Shortly thereafter, other manufacturers followed suit. Side airbags became available about 10-15 years later. The US Department of Transportation estimates that use of airbags save about 3,000 Americans per year, while the additional use of seatbelts saved an additional 12,000 lives per year.

Inflatable evacuation chutes have been on commercial airlines since the 1960s. Early chutes could be punctured by spiked high heels worn by women. While this is less of a problem with today's chutes, women are advised to remove these shoes to avoid ankle sprains when sliding down the chute and hitting the ground.

There have been no toxicities reported due to ruptured air bags following automobile accidents. The amount of sodium azide is much smaller than what would be in an airplane chute. There has been accidental deployment of evacuation chutes when doors were opened by flight attendants prior to disarming the evacuation chute. This is the reason that flight attendants remind each other to "disarm doors and cross check."

Unrelated to air bags, there have been a few other cases of sodium azide exposures including six Harvard professors in 2009, and patrons eating at a restaurant in Dallas a year later. While none died, they were dizzy and hypotensive.

Hospital Daycare

****

Deepa's family was originally from Mumbai, India. Her father was an electrical engineer who received his master's degree in the United States. Shortly after finishing his studies, her dad moved his family to the West Coast. Deepa was seven at the time. Like many first-generation immigrants, she struggled with her cultural identity. She cherished her Indian heritage, but very much wanted to be just like any other American kid. When Deepa was eighteen, her parents arranged a date for her with an Indian boy. He was in the same caste as her family. She resented her family's interference, but eventually fell in love with Javender. By the time she was 21, Deepa was married to Javender, who was two years older than she was.

Like his father-in-law, Javender was also an engineer. But he was much more ambitious. He grew impatient working for a computer hardware company. So after three years, Javender left the company, and with a classmate from college, they formed their own Internet company. They provided digital tools that helped the Bollywood industry in making animated movies. Javender spent most of his time starting up the business, with frequent trips back to Mumbai. He had little time for Deepa.

Deepa became pregnant when she was 25. By then, Javender's business had taken off, and he was spending even less time at home. Deepa began to resent her husband but felt that there was nothing she could do about it. So when baby Seema arrived, Deepa hoped that her new daughter would give her renewed purpose. At first, life was good again for Deepa. She knew that Seema was totally dependent on her and that made her feel wanted. However, by the time she hit the "terrible twos," Seema was wild and uncontrollable. She would have loud temper tantrums, throwing food around the house, and could not be reasoned with. Deepa could see that Seema was much like her father, very independent and needing to have her own way. Seema became more of a burden to Deepa and she started to resent her daughter for it. *Maybe if I had a career*, she thought to herself, *I would have motivation in my life again*. Javender's business was doing well and they could afford a nanny. So in the fall, Deepa enrolled in the community college as a pharmacy student.

*

One of my jobs at the General was teaching students the basic principles of poisons. In the School of Pharmacy, I had a core block of lectures that dealt with different types of poisonings, including heavy metals like arsenic, anticoagulants such as rat poisons, mushroom intoxicants, analgesics, and toxic alcohols, such as methanol and ethylene glycol. The course also contained a laboratory component where students learned about atomic absorption spectroscopy and gas chromatography, the equipment used to detect these poisons. Deepa was one of my students. She was top in her class. Unlike the other students whose attention would drift from time to time, Deepa wrote copious notes and often stayed after class to ask questions. She asked me one that I thought was strange.

"How much methanol or ethylene glycol could be given to make someone sick but not necessarily kill them?"

I responded jokingly, "Why, are you trying to get rid of someone?"

Deepa laughed and then said, "No, just curious. Never mind, forget I asked that question."

*

About seven months later, a 2 and a half year old Indian child was admitted to the General Hospital with severe metabolic acidosis. This is a serious, life-threatening condition that must be treated immediately. In addition to a diabetic crisis and septic shock, poisons are included in the differential diagnosis of this type of acidosis. A negative ketone ruled out diabetic ketoacidosis and a negative lactate and lack of a fever made sepsis less likely. So the medical team suspected a toxic alcohol, such as ethylene glycol or antifreeze. Ethylene glycol is much more poisonous than ethyl alcohol. Because these poisonings are infrequent, my lab did not offer tests for them at the time, so instead, samples were sent to a reference lab that used gas chromatography. The report showed an exceptionally high concentration of ethylene glycol in the urine of the child. This level would have killed most adults but this child appeared to be tolerant.

I found out about this case from my resident who was asked for approval to perform the glycol test. Given the unusual circumstances, I went to the pediatric intensive care unit to see this child. Much to my astonishment, when I arrived, I found my former student in the room with the child.

"Deepa, what are you doing here?" I asked. Then I realized that she was the mother of the patient that I came to see.

"This is my daughter, Seema," Deepa said. "She is really sick. Professor, how could this have happened?" I was going to ask Deepa the exact same question. "You must help her," she said. "She's all that I have." I assured her that Seema was in the best of hands.

Deepa went on to ask, "Can the hospital keep her here for as long as possible? She is better off here than at home." This last comment disturbed me. It is well known that hospitals are not very safe places for children; hospital-acquired infections are a major problem.

Why did she say that?" I wondered. *Was there some abuse going on at home?* Without answering her question, I said I had to check on other patients and left the room. I rushed to see the intensive care pediatrician in charge of Seema's care.

*

Dr. John Reynolds had been the Director of our Pediatric ICU for more than 20 years. He had seen a lot of pediatric poisonings, but this case was a new one. Accidental poisonings of a toddler by ethylene glycol were extremely rare. A review of Seema's medical record showed that she had been admitted multiple times for the same medical problem: a failure to thrive and too much acid in her blood. It first started when Seema was switched from breast milk and baby formula to baby food. In each case, Seema responded to treatment and was sent home after a few days.

When Deepa could not provide an explanation as to how her child was exposed to ethylene glycol, Dr. Reynolds contacted the state's child protective services. The team performed a thorough questioning of Seema's parents and her caregivers. They sent an investigative team to Deepa and Javender's home. In the refrigerator, they found a baby bottle with a small amount of milk in it. It was confiscated and sent to the same lab that had tested Seema's urine. The bottle contents contained formula without any contaminations. However, when the lab tested the nipple, it contained trace amounts of ethylene glycol. I then told Dr. Reynolds that Deepa was one of my former pharmacy students, and that she'd learned about toxic alcohol poisonings through my lectures. I also told him of Deepa's question about the amount it would take to make someone sick. I never dreamed that one of my own students would use this knowledge to poison her own child. Confronted with the evidence, Deepa denied having poisoned Seema.

"I love my child and would never do anything to harm her."

"What was the ethylene glycol doing in her baby bottle?" the child protective services investigator asked. Deepa had no answer for that.

Dr. Hans Sinclair, a forensic psychiatrist was brought in to review the case. After meeting with Deepa, the psychiatrist concluded that she was suffering from Munchausen syndrome by proxy, a psychiatric disease characterized by people purposely causing harm to their children. The disease occurs almost exclusively in women. The men in the relationship are often disengaged in the rearing of their children.

"Deepa was overwhelmed by the needs of Seema, and needed to find a way to get out of her responsibility," explained Dr. Sinclair. "So she poisoned her child until she was so sick that she had to be cared for in a hospital."

Given the evidence against Deepa, the district attorney's office filed criminal charges against her. Although she protested that she was innocent, Deepa was convicted of child endangerment. She was sentenced to a psychiatric facility where she would receive regular psychiatric care. As Javender had no involvement with the poisonings, Seema was remanded to his custody. Under his care, Seema appeared to be better, although she continued to be very small for her age and was sick more often than not.

Javender learned all he could about Munchausen syndrome by proxy. He realized that his wife was sick and needed professional help. He regularly visited Deepa in the facility and occasionally brought Seema. So that he could be a full-time father, Javender turned over the day-to-day operations of his company to his partner. After a few months, Deepa felt better with the medications she was given. The couple was granted conjugal visits. Within six months, Deepa became pregnant again. While at the psychiatric facility, Deepa gave birth to a healthy baby boy; they named him Vijay. The child lived with Javender and his family. They would bring him to see Deepa while she was in prison. Within a year, Vijay developed a pattern of sickness that was very similar to what happened with Seema, including several episodes of metabolic acidosis. He made several trips to the emergency department but the doctors could never find out what was wrong. During one hospital visit, Javender came to me for help. He never blamed me for my role in Deepa's conviction. He told me that he and Deepa had another child and that this boy was having medical problems similar to what Seema had undergone. Thinking that the illnesses of these two siblings might be related genetically, I asked the family to provide a fresh urine sample from Vijay for genetic testing. We now offered a lab test for congenital diseases. This test also detected methanol and ethylene glycol. When I got the data from the lab and reviewed it, my jaw dropped. A terrible mistake had been made.

I called Javender and asked for a fresh urine sample from Seema. After this specimen was tested, I was now certain that something had gone wrong. I went into the lab's archival records for the original urine test report on Seema. To my surprise, the sample had not been sent to the hospital's normal reference lab. Then I remembered that a few years ago, our hospital administrators wanted all specialty tests sent to a new reference lab because they were less expensive. This "experiment" of using a low cost provider only lasted a few months because the quality of the lab was questioned on several occasions. The company folded a few months later. I had forgotten that we'd sent samples to this lab years ago. I gathered the facts and called Dr. John Reynolds to explain my findings.

"I have proof that the original lab that tested Seema's urine sample made an egregious error," I explained. "It turns out that Seema's urine contained propionic acid and not ethylene glycol. This acid is excreted in the urine of patients with propionic acidemia, a congenital disease. These children lack a critical enzyme needed to break down fat and fatty acids in the body. Acidosis begins with a high protein diet," I continued. "We use chromatography to separate the compounds, and have found that both ethylene glycol and propionic acid have similar appearances on the chromatogram. To the untrained eye, one can be confused for the other. Since ethylene glycol poisoning is more common than propionic acidemia, the lab we used back then, which was not experienced with the limitations of liquid chromatographic testing for metabolic diseases, made the wrong conclusion. The lab didn't use mass spectrometry as a detector, which would have told them what was really present.

Still puzzled, Dr. Reynolds asked, "So what tipped you off to go back and look at Seema's original results?"

"It was really Vijay, Seema's new baby brother that made me suspicious," I said. "He has the same history of multiple presentations of acidosis coupled with a failure to thrive. In this case, however, Deepa was in custody and could not have poisoned her son. And we never thought Javender was involved since he was always so busy. So I looked elsewhere for an explanation."

Reynolds then said, "But what about the baby bottle that contained ethylene glycol?"

"My best guess is that the baby bottle nipple contained Seemas' saliva. The trace amount of propionic acid found in her saliva was also erroneously detected by the lab."

Reynolds sighed and finally said, "So Deepa was telling the truth after all? You know, she never wavered in proclaiming her innocence. Now that we know, we can manage Seema and Vijay's illnesses much better. And we need to get Deepa home to be with her children."

Armed with the truth, Dr. Reynolds got the courts to reexamine the evidence against Deepa. Both Dr. Reynolds and I testified on her behalf. Fresh urine from both children was retested by an independent laboratory to verify my finding of propionic acid. After a re-trial, Deepa was acquitted of the charge of child endangerment, released from the facility, and returned to her family. Her three-year ordeal was over; she had not been using the hospital as daycare for Seema after all. Deepa and Javender were never bitter about what happened to them. It was a series of mistakes that began with an erroneous lab report. They were just glad that they now were all together for the first time as a real family.

Now that propionic acidemia was diagnosed in both Seema and Vijay, the appropriate treatment was given to both children. This included a protein-restricted diet and carnitine supplementation to maintain energy stores. Although these children continued to get sick more often than normal, their health improved after these measures were taken. Javender realized that he had neglected his wife and family in order to have a successful career. But they were still young and had a lifetime ahead of them. Javender sold his business to his partner and became an employee and stockholder of the company. When he went home each night, he stopped thinking about his job, something he couldn't have done before. He curtailed his traveling to India to just once every other year, and took Deepa and the kids with him.

*

Munchausen syndrome is defined as harm caused by oneself. It was first recognized as a disease entity in the mid-19th century. A variant form, Munchausen syndrome "by proxy," is when the harm is caused by a loved one, most often the mother. Both are recognized psychiatric disorders. The term Munchausen was coined in 1951 by Dr. Richard Asher, an eminent British endocrinologist. The syndrome is named after Baron von Münchausen, an 18th century Prussian officer, who fabricated stories about his military exploits. Munchausen by proxy was first described in

1976. There are no established databases that document the true number of Munchausen by proxy cases per year, although annual estimates in the United States range from 200 to 1200 cases. Boys are equally affected as girls. The average age of the affected child at the time of diagnosis is about 4 years.

I regretted my role in suggesting to Deepa's pediatrician that Deepa caused harm to her first-born child. As it turned out, she was innocent and I jumped to the wrong conclusion. Fortunately, I was able to play a major role in restoring the child back to the family. It is important for me and my employees in the clinical laboratory to understand that there are people – and significant consequences – behind the results we produce.

Duffer Dysfunction

****

Carl Roper learned how to play golf while caddying at his father's country club, Piedmont Greens. When not on a bag for a client, he and the other caddies would spend hours at the driving range and putting greens after school and on weekends. Back then, woods were really made of wood, and if you hit the ball wrong with an iron, it would cut a permanent dent into the ball. Carl's parents were happy that he spent time at the club, because it kept him occupied and out of trouble. By the time Carl was twelve years old, the local pro noticed that Carl had a natural swing and could drive a ball 220 yards. The pro gave him tips on pitching and putting, and encouraged him to play competitively. Within two years, Carl won the club's junior golf championship, beating kids that were as much as five years older than him. Carl joined his high school golf team and even as a freshman, was the best golfer on the team. In his senior year, Carl won the individual championship for the entire state. He received several scholarships to play college golf and enrolled at the State University. During his sophomore year, he led his team to the NCAA championship. Carl was the tournament's individual champion, having shot an amazing nine under par. At this point, Carl was at a crossroads in his career. There was nothing more to accomplish while playing amateur golf. His old golf mentor at

Piedmont Greens told him that it was time for him to join the professional ranks. Carl hesitated because he really enjoyed the social life at college. He was in a fraternity and was dating more than his share of college co-eds. In the end, he decided to go for the money and left school.

Despite his success in college, Carl was just a marginal golfer throughout his career on the Professional Golf Association Tour. The best players during his time were Jack Nicklaus, Lee Trevino, Tom Watson, and also Arnold Palmer, whose career was then in its later years. While Carl never won a major tournament, he did manage to win a few of the smaller ones and finished near the top in some others. He played in the pre-Tiger Woods era, before the million dollar purses. Nevertheless, Carl's earnings were sufficient to sustain him on the tour for the better part of 20 years.

Being on the road during most of the year, Carl's social life was linked to his golf profession. He dated women that he met at tournaments or who worked at country clubs where events were held. Some of them would leave their telephone numbers and hotel keys for him. Carl took advantage of his notoriety as a pro athlete and had "one-night stands" with many of these women. He waited until he was in his early thirties before he got married to a pretty girl who managed a snack bar at one of the courses. By then, Carl's ranking began to decline and he started drinking more regularly. Unfortunately, the marriage only lasted two years. Citing neglect and emotional distress, his ex-wife got a generous award from the divorce. Three years later, he married another woman with no connection to golf; she was a barmaid at his favorite tavern. Carl stopped drinking for a few years and his golf game improved. He and his new wife tried to have a baby. But they were unsuccessful in conceiving after several years, and their failure ultimately led to his second divorce.

Carl left the professional tour at the age of 42. He was no longer competitive and wasn't winning enough money to sustain his travel expenses. But he wanted to stay in the game, so he became a teaching professional at his father's old country club. Since he'd started there as a boy, he became somewhat of a legend at the club and they were happy to put him on the payroll. For a while, this satisfied his golf needs for many years. Carl wasn't big on teaching children. His preference was attractive middle-aged wealthy women. He had affairs with many of them. It was safe because he knew none of these women would leave their rich husbands. He would back off if he sensed a woman wanted more than just casual sex.

After seven years on the job at Piedmont Greens, Carl was becoming bored with teaching. He yearned for his competitive life again. Since he was turning 50 soon, he decided to make a run on the PGA's Senior Tour. Having switched from wood to the modern alloy-metal drivers, Carl now could drive a ball as far as he did when he was on the regular tour, and farther than most of the pros on the senior PGA tour. So he spent the rest of the year training. He hired a coach and did well in several tournaments on the Nationwide Tour. This professional tour is a notch below the regular PGA tour. The next year, Carl got golf exemptions based on his prior performances on the regular tour, which enabled him to enter tournaments on the senior tour. As before, Carl was competitive and won some money on this tour. Even more important to him was that he was able to stay connected to the best of the game and, at the same time, conquer new female targets.

When Carl turned 55, he was not able to perform in the bedroom as well as before. While his sexual appetite was still strong, he sometimes failed to get aroused at the right moment. He went to his doctor to see if there was anything that could be done therapeutically. His doctor considered giving him a prescription for Viagra. However, because Carl developed hypertension, he was told that this drug might not be safe for him. Carl left the office depressed. Old age was interfering with his sex life. Then one day, at an airport on his way to a tournament, he noticed a magazine ad that piqued his interest: *Treat erectile dysfunction using Trojan, an herbal medication containing only natural substances.* Once he got to San Francisco for the tournament, Carl went to a store that sold nutritional supplements and bought a supply of Trojan. He had a date with Jill, one of the women who worked at the registration table at the tournament; he would test out the herb that night.

Trojan came in clear unmarked capsules. Inside the capsules, he could see some green, grainy materials quite unlike the powders that were found in normal therapeutic drugs. He swallowed two pills a few minutes before knocking on Jill's hotel room door. Jill let him in; she was wearing a black negligee. Carl was excited and got an erection almost immediately. Their sex was better than any Carl had in many years.

This stuff really works, he said to himself. After sex, he fell asleep, although he still had an erection. The next morning, Jill woke up with Carl next to her.

She shook him, "Carl, get up. You have to play today.

Get up." But there was no response. She pulled back the covers, but still, Carl did not move and could not be awakened. She then noticed that he was still erect. Jill was learned that this was rigor mortis. She shrieked and called the hotel operator for help. Carl had made his last stroke.

*

Carl's body was positioned face up on a gurney and was wheeled into the medical examiner's office. He was covered with a sheet with only his toes and an identification tag exposed. Around his torso, there was a protrusion that formed a mini-tent with the sheet. Herbert and Ernest the dieners who assist medical examiners with autopsies had a field day with this sight. Levity can be very therapeutic when working daily with death. Over the years, they'd seen more than their share of murders, child molestations, rape victims, horribly disfiguring injuries, and various stages of human body decomposition. It definitely takes a special type of individual to do this type of work year in and year out. So when a case like this came in, they couldn't resist.

"He forgot to put his putter away," Herbert said to Ernest.

"That's not a putter, that's one of those long brush tees used for 450 cc titanium drivers," said Ernest, who was an avid golfer.

"But he forgot to tee up the ball; two of them are still on the ground and...."

Then they heard their boss entering the room. Both Herbert and Ernest were wearing green surgical scrubs as pants. They looked at each other and nonverbally agreed to untie their scrub strings at the waistline.

The medical examiner arrived and said, "Knock it off guys, and get back to work." He heard the jokes they were making at the decedent's expense.

"Yes sir!" they both said in unison, standing tall and erect, while saluting their boss. Their scrubs fell from their waist and onto their ankles exposing their boxer shorts. The pathologist couldn't help himself; he broke rank and laughed out loud. He needed some humor in his day, also*

*

I got the call a few days later from the medical examiner. "We just did an autopsy on a guy who died of a heart attack. There were some unmarked herbal pills in his pocket. We're wondering if this could have contributed to his death. Can you take a look at the pills?"

"Sure," I said to the pathologist. "Anything else I should know about?"

"Yes, he died with a penile erection, which is highly unusual. And he was a professional golfer."

Postmortem blood and urine samples came to my lab the next day along with the pills he allegedly took. "This is a job for our high-resolution mass spectrometer," I instructed one of my techs, who went to work. "The medical examiner suspects that the herbal pills were adulterated with designer erectile dysfunction drugs. While the active ingredients of Viagra and Cialis are regulated by the Food and Drug Administration, herbal medications are considered nutritional supplements and are not regulated."

"So what are we looking for?" Betsy, my tech, asked.

"Drug analogs to tadalafel and sildenafil, the real drugs

that are contained within Cialis and Viagra, respectively." She took the samples from me and went into the lab.

About three hours later, I got a call. "Professor, we've found something very interesting in both the blood sample and medication." I left my office and went downstairs to the lab where the testing was being conducted.

When I arrived, Betsy said, "We have molecular weight matches for two compounds, hydroxyhomosildenafil and acetildenafil. Is this what you're looking for, Professor?"

When I looked at the data, it appeared to be consistent with the statements made to me by the medical examiner. "But we don't have a standard, so I have to be sure. Let's go on the Internet and see if we can purchase these chemicals."

When I got back to the office, I could not find a source for acetildenafil. There was a listing for a manufacturer of hydroxyhomosidenafil in China. I sent them an email and received a reply the next day: "The list price is $1000 US. The minimum purchase quantity is 100 kilograms or 200 pounds."

"But we don't need that much to standardize our instrument. One milligram would be more than enough," Betsy said.

"I know, but they don't know we're an analytical testing laboratory. They probably wouldn't sell it to us if they knew how we were using it. They think we are an herbal manufacturer and that we're going to spike our erectile dysfunction products with this chemical. We have no choice but to buy this large quantity."

"Don't you be using this stuff," Betsy warned me, jokingly.

"Very funny," I laughed. Let's not get too personal!"

When the drug came in, we did some analytical procedures to determine its mass and purity. We found that it was largely free of contaminants. "Since it is meant for human consumption, they did a good job of removing impurities," I said to Betsy. "Let's see what drug levels we find in our old duffer."

When the analysis was complete, I called the medical examiner to report our findings. "The herbal that Mr. Roper took was something called Trojan. This herbal contains two different Viagra-like chemical analogs. We also analyzed some prescription pills of both Cialis and Viagra and compared the results against Trojan. While I don't know the relative potency of sildenafil and its analogs, it appears that Mr. Roper had an excessive amount of drug present in his blood and urine. I suspect this had an important role in his heart attack."

Carl's death in his hotel room hit the sporting news. He was well known to the golfing world, but it was back-page news to the more important new stories that day. While the postmortem results were a matter of public record, nobody mentioned that he had taken an erectile drug and was having sex just before he died. It was reported as just a heart attack. Piedmont Greens named their club championship after Carl Roper. His picture hangs in the pro shop over a plaque inscribed with the dates of his birth and his death.

*

This case demonstrates the dangers of taking herbal medications from unreliable sources. The notion that natural substances are safe must be dispelled, as there are many compounds found in nature that are toxic. Moreover, in order to cash in on the current popularity of homeopathic remedies, clandestine laboratories are adulterating their products with real drugs and drug analogs and marketing them to a non-suspecting public.

Herbal medications and natural supplements are widely used throughout America. Because they are defined as "nutraceuticals," they are considered safe and are not regulated by the Food and Drug Administration. However, some herbal products are not "all natural" as advertised. In order to achieve the desired medical indications, these concoctions may be adulterated with drugs or drug analogs to prescription medications. The presence of these substances is not disclosed on herbal labeling. Manufacturers of herbals may not practice good manufacturing techniques, and the concentration of the active ingredients might vary from lot to lot.

After Carl Roper's death, I submitted a complaint to the California branch of the FDA regarding Trojan and the ingredients that I'd found in the herbal. This triggered an investigation regarding the safety of this product. Letters were sent to the manufacturer asking for documentation of their manufacturing practices. The company, located in southern China, did not respond. In the meantime, a recall was distributed to retail outlets to remove Trojan products from their shelves. Learning of the recall, the manufacturer closed their shop and the product was no longer produced. It is very likely, however, that the individuals involved have reopened at a new manufacturing location and that the product has been re-introduced under a different label. Due to the lack of FDA surveillance, this is a situation that truly warrants the warning of "buyer beware."

Toadstool Gourmand

****

Mei-Tse Chang was a 64-year old mother of two sons and grandmother of five. She had lived most of her life in Taiwan, but after her husband died, Mei lived in Taipei with her son Tad and his family during the fall and winter, and in Berkeley California with her son Goh and his family during the spring and summer.

"I can't stand the summer months in Taiwan anymore," she told Tad. "The hot and humid weather never used to bother me, but I guess I'm getting old and can't take the heat."

Tad and Goh were both successful businessmen. Tad owned a silicon chip factory in Taiwan and Goh was co-owner of a software development company in California. Mei did not mind the 14-hour flight each way because her sons would book her in first class, where the seats reclined completely. If she wasn't sleeping, she would pass the time reading or knitting something for the grandchildren. Tad had three daughters, and Goh had twin 8 year-old boys, Nelson and Pang.

Mei arrived for her stay in Berkeley shortly after one of the wettest springs the Bay Area had seen in years. The conditions were ideal for the growth of wild mushrooms. One night, Goh and his wife Hua were to attend a business dinner. They asked Mei to babysit for the twins. She told them she would make her specialty dish, fresh mushroom chicken noodle stir-fry. Normally, she would go to the farmers market on a Sunday and pick up a variety of mushrooms. This time, though, she told Goh that she would take the boys out to the field near Goh's house and pick fresh ones for this special meal. Hua was a little leery of Mei cooking wild mushrooms and expressed her concern privately to Goh. But Goh assured Hua that his mother had been picking mushrooms in Taiwan for many years and was sort of a toadstool expert. So Hua didn't say anything further even though the idea of Mei picking fresh mushrooms for dinner still made her nervous. It was difficult for a young wife to challenge a mother-in-law in the Asian culture, especially someone like Mei who had a dominant personality. Hua spent most of her life in the United States but still respected her Asian culture. She would later regret her reluctance to speak up that night.

Mei and the twins went out to the field carrying a cloth-lined wicker basket and picked a few dozen mushrooms. "Back home, we call these mushrooms căogū," she told the boys. "They are very good eating. Let's go home and I'll start cooking." And they gathered their baskets and headed home.

Back home, Mei washed the mushrooms carefully, sliced them vertically into thin slices, and put them into a wok. She then added the other ingredients for the dish: cooked chicken, broth, shallots, thick Japanese udon noodles, and spices. She turned the burner on high to heat the wok, adding sesame oil and soy sauce. When everything was fully cooked, Mei served the meal. Having been out all afternoon in the field picking mushrooms with their *ni-ni*, the twins were especially hungry and had second helpings. After dinner, they all settled down in the living room. Mei turned on the television, and the boys were playing video games on their Game Boys.

Within a few hours, the twins developed nausea and complained of gastrointestinal cramping. Nelson seemed to have been hit the hardest. He was moaning and doubled over with pain. Mei put both boys to bed and called her son. Goh and Hua were having their coffee and dessert when the call came in.

"The kids aren't feeling well, and neither am I," Mei told Goh. "What should I do?" Hua overheard the conversation and uncharacteristically grabbed the phone from her husband.

"What symptoms do they have, Mom?"

"Stomach cramps," Mei replied.

Hua got up and said, "We're leaving now," as she hung up Goh's phone. She then turned to her husband and said, "Goh, they might have been poisoned by the mushrooms." They thanked their hosts, told them of their family emergency, and left immediately. When they arrived home, Hua ran into the house. Mei was lying down on the living room sofa.

"Where are the twins?" Hua asked.

"In bed," Mei replied. Hua rushed into the boys' room just as Goh was entering the front door. Once inside her sons' room, Hua saw that they were both curled up on their beds, moaning.

Pang said, "Mom, we feel terrible. Make it go away." Hua felt Nelson's forehead. No fever.

Then Nelson said, "I'm having trouble breathing, Mom." She went over to his bed and saw that he was laboring to breathe while lying in a fetal position.

Just then, Goh entered the room. Hua shouted at him,

"Call 9-1-1 right now! Our kids are really sick. We need to go to the ER. How is Mom? Does she have the same problems?"

"She's sick too," Goh replied as he punched in the emergency number.

Within 10 minutes, help arrived. The paramedics took Mei and the two boys to the emergency department of the General Hospital. Goh and Hua followed the ambulance in their car. The patients were immediately triaged into beds. The triage nurse asked the parents what happened. Hua told the nurse that her mother-in-law picked fresh mushrooms that afternoon which she'd used in their dinner and she suspected that they might have been poisonous. The nurse relayed the information to the emergency department team. When it was clear that this was a case of mushroom poisoning, the patients were admitted and transported to intensive care units. Mei went to the medical ICU and the two boys went to the pediatric ICU. Both of the boys were sedated and intubated because of their respiratory issues. Intravenous lines were established and each boy was hooked up to a solution of lactated ringers, a solution of electrolytes and glucose. Blood was collected and sent to the clinical laboratory for electrolytes, blood gases, and liver and renal function tests.

Dr. Todd Goldman was paged. He was a hepatologist and the resident expert in mushroom poisonings. Over the years, Dr. Goldman had treated many other cases of mushroom poisoning and was conducting clinical research on new therapeutic modalities. He just finished his own dinner with his wife at a restaurant — ironically, a dish containing shiitake mushrooms. When he got the page, Dr. Goldman told his wife that there was an emergency at the hospital. He paid the bill, put

217

her into a cab, and rushed over to the hospital. She was used to this routine; the price of being a doctor's spouse. Dr. Goldman arrived at the hospital, put his "Emergency Department MD" sign on his car's dashboard, and rushed in. He went to the pediatric ICU first, knowing that children were at greater risk for death than adults. Hua and Goh were in the waiting room, obviously distressed.

Dr. Goldman disinfected his hands with the hand sanitizer dispenser on the wall near the PICU door and went in to see the boys. He then went to see their grandmother in the MICU. After that he returned to the PICU waiting room to speak with the parents. "Are any of the mushrooms still available at home?" he asked them. "If we can identify them, it might alter our treatment strategy."

Goh told his wife, "You stay here; I'll go home right now to see what I can find." Hua agreed. She was in no condition to drive anyway as she was so upset. Goh drove to the house and ran into the kitchen. He knew his mother used the wok for cooking the dish. He was not surprised to find that the kitchen was spotless. The wok and all dishes were washed and hanging in the drying rack. He opened the refrigerator to see if there were any leftover noodles. He found only the kid's spaghetti from last night's dinner. He then looked around the cabinets and counters, not exactly sure what he was looking for. He then spotted the wicker basket. It still had a few residual pieces of mushrooms. There were no intact mushrooms. He grabbed the basket, covered the pieces with the cloth, and rushed back to the hospital.

When he arrived back at the PICU, Hua asked, "What

did you find at home?"

Goh showed her what he found and said, "There isn't a lot here. I'm not sure it will be helpful in identifying what kind of mushrooms Mom picked." Hua told him that Dr. Goldman was now examining Mei in the MICU and that he should go there. When he arrived, he found Dr. Goldman examining Mei. Goh showed him the tiny mushroom pieces that were remaining in the basket.

"Not much to go on here," the doctor remarked. "But I'll call the clinical laboratory and see if there is something that can be done." With that, Dr. Goldman called the head of the chemistry laboratory at the General.

I had worked with Dr. Goldman before on mushroom poisonings. In anticipation of future mushroom poisoning cases and at the advice of Dr. Goldman, we worked out a mushroom toxin testing procedure called the Meixner Test. The majority of human mushroom poisonings are caused by consuming the *Amanita phalloides* mushroom. The Meixner Test involves squeezing mushrooms and allowing a drop of juice to fall onto common newsprint. Newspapers and telephone books contain lignin, an integral part of plant cell walls including wood pulp. In the presence of a drop of acid, a blue color reaction on the newsprint is caused by a reaction between lignin and α-amatoxin, the poison found in *Amanita*. I took the mushroom pieces given to them by Goh and performed the test. It was positive for amatoxin. Grandmother inadvertently poisoned herself and her grandchildren. I called Dr. Goldman and told him that indeed *Amanita phalloides* was the poison in question.

In the meantime, both the boys and their grandmother

took a turn for the worse, not surprising in light of the liver function test results just returned from my lab. Dr. Goldman met with Hua and Goh to discuss the therapeutic plan. "We have confirmed that your family has eaten poisonous mushrooms."

"How could that have happened?" Goh asked. "My mother has been harvesting mushrooms in Taiwan for years. She knows what is poisonous and what is not."

"In Taiwan," Dr. Goldman said, "there is a species of mushrooms called *Volvariella volvacea*. It is used widely in East and Southeast Asia. It is not poisonous, but it looks very much like *Amanita*...."

"Never mind, it doesn't matter now how it happened," Hua interrupted. Goh had never seen her so demonstrative. "How are my boys doing now?"

"The twins and their grandmother have early signs of liver failure," Dr. Goldman explained. "The aminotransferase enzymes are increased. If this progresses to complete liver failure, the only measure is an emergency liver transplantation. That option will be subject to the availability of a donor organ. There are more people who need a liver than the number of organs available."

Hua started crying.

"There is one other hope, "Dr. Goldman continued. "In Europe, mushroom poisoning is more common than it is here. They have been experimenting with a therapy based on milk thistle and had some early successes. Milk thistle is a plant native to the Mediterranean. The name comes from the fact that the plant contains a milky sap and the leaves have white blotches. It is a natural remedy for liver disease. The active ingredient is silymarin. It works on mushroom poisoning by accelerating the clearance of amatoxin through the bile circulation. But it only works if it is given before there is a substantial amount of liver injury. There is nothing silly about the healing properties of silymarin," Dr. Goldman remarked.

"Doctor, what does this mean for our family?" Goh asked, sounding desperate and a little impatient.

Dr. Goldman continued, "Unfortunately, this antidote has not been approved in the U.S. But I called the emergency number at the FDA this evening and asked for their permission to have some milk thistle sent to us under their "Emergency Investigational Drug" provision. They were reluctant at first, saying that the data was unproven. I've seen the data and I believe it only lacks statistical power. I mean, there just haven't yet been enough patients where this medication has been used. So I pleaded with them and said that the life of two little boys and their grandmother was literally in their hands. My request for special permission was granted."

Goh and Hua nodded their heads slightly at these last, somewhat hopeful words.

The doctor went on, "But then I had to find someone who had a stock of this medication and was willing to send me what we needed. Fortunately, I know a pharmacist in Italy. He was home in bed but he got up and rushed to his hospital. The milk thistle is now on an Alitalia flight from Rome and will be here tomorrow morning. We can only hope for the best moving forward."

The next morning, the "milk man" arrived from the airport with his priceless cargo. Dr. Goldman had one of his residents wait at the airport baggage area to retrieve it. He rushed it to the PICU where Dr. Goldman was waiting. When he opened the package, he saw that there were only 12 vials instead of the 18 that he was expecting. "Oh no," he exclaimed to his resident. "We need six vials for each patient. We only have enough for two of them. If we tried to split the supply up three ways, it might not work for any of them."

A family meeting was called. Dr. Goldman contacted another colleague and more milk thistle was on its way. But there would be another 12-hour delay. In the meantime, they had to decide who was going to get the initial doses.

"Nelson is the sickest right now. We need to do something immediately," Dr. Goldman said without hesitation. "I'm leaning toward Pang to receive the other dose because children are affected by amatoxin poisons more so than adults. But you have to be okay with this difficult decision."

There was no question in Hua's mind which person should get the other half of the medication. "It was her fault that they are here now!" she shouted at Goh. "I told you that I was not comfortable with her using these mushrooms, but you said it would be okay. If either of them dies, I will never ever forgive you!" She ran out of the room, tears streaming down her cheeks.

Goh had to make the most difficult decision of his life. How could he choose between his mother and his child? Dr. Goldman sat down with Goh. Hua came back to the waiting room. Dr. Goldman told him that mushrooms were more poisonous for children than adults. Goh called his brother in Taiwan for his advice. He had been updating Tad every step of the way. Tad said that he would support whatever decision they made. While he hoped his mother could survive, he didn't want it to be at the expense of one of his young nephews. So they decided that they needed to treat both boys with the thistle and hope that either a liver would become available for their mom, or that she could survive until the next shipment of thistle arrived.

The two boys did well with the milk thistle. They would not need a transplant and were able to go home after two weeks in the hospital. The second shipment of thistle arrived the next day, but by then, the extent of Mei's liver injury was too great. There was no liver transplant available to her. She survived for a few more days before she died. Goh felt tremendous guilt for the decision they made.

Goh arranged for his mother's body to be flown to Taiwan so that she could be buried next to her husband. He and his family flew in to attend Mei's funeral. Many of Mei's friends came. Tad assembled pictures of his mother and father and had a slide show during the funeral service. One by one, the visitors walked by to pay their final respects, eventually leaving only Tad, Goh, and their families. The twins were the last ones to approach their grandmother's casket. They stood in front, bowed three times, and gently placed inside one rose apiece.

*

In 2010, of the 358 people in California who were treated with mushroom poisoning, one person died and 16 others spent time in an intensive care unit, according to the California Poison Control Center. Five required a liver transplant. Milk thistle is still not FDA-cleared for use in the United States to prevent liver failure induced by amatoxin mushroom poisoning. One manufacturer has initiated a clinical trial that will enable emergency access to this antidote for poisoned patients.

This is not a randomized trial of thistle vs. placebo, so everyone over the age of two can potentially benefit. However, the therapeutic value of milk thistle remains to be determined. While too late for Mei-Tse Chang, this may be a life-saving alternative to liver transplantation and it may save the lives of future mushroom-poisoned patients.

Jacked!

****

During high school, all of Jimmy Smith's friends called him a gym rat, someone who was always working out. It started when he was in junior high, when he was picked on by the older kids in the neighborhood. When he got home after being roughed up by these kids, his father, Jerome, a retired African American U.S. Marine Corp veteran, would say to Jimmy, "Tough it out, kid. I don't want a wuss living in my house!" Jimmy's mother, who was Caucasian, wanted to protect her only son, but Jerome told her not to interfere. "This will make him strong," he said.

Seeing that he wasn't going to get any sympathy from his parents, Jimmy decided very early in life to take matters into his own hands. That was the start of him becoming a workout fanatic. When he was 14, he bought a pair of dumbbells and started doing arm curls on his own at home. He was a scrawny kid and didn't want the other kids to see him exercising. Jimmy didn't think he would enjoy working out, and he didn't at first. His muscles were sore during the first week, and he could barely lift his arms above his head. Even after two weeks, he saw no improvement in his biceps, so he almost gave up. But there was a girl at school whom he liked, and this motivated him to continue. After two months, he felt the weight training was finally paying off. He had more energy and he gained a few pounds. His body also began to mature. As his confidence grew, he began working out in the high school's weight room. There, he met other boys who worked out regularly. Several of the older kids befriended him. They taught him how to use the lifting machines, spotted him when he was working out with free weights, and encouraged him to press more pounds.

During one of these sessions, a weightlifting friend told Jimmy about dietary supplements. "Man, if you want to really bulk up, you should try this stuff," he said. Jimmy was directed to a general nutrition store, where he bought products that contained creatine, glutamine, branched chain amino acids, and proteins. He also found out about anabolic steroids and bought them through the mail without telling his parents. But shortly after starting, he developed severe acne on his face and back. His parents thought it was just because he was going through puberty. Jimmy read that the anabolic steroids can produces zits as a side effect, so he stopped taking them after a year.

Over 18 months, Jimmy gained 25 pounds of muscle, and nobody at school picked on him anymore. He became one of the bigger kids. His parents noticed a change in Jimmy's demeanor. He told them that when he graduated from high school, he was going to enlist in the Marine Corp. His mother was hoping he would choose college instead, but his father was proud that his son was following in his footsteps. On his eighteenth birthday, Jimmy got a tattoo in Chinese characters on each of his now very large biceps. The Chinese character on the right side supposedly meant "pumped." The left bicep tat was intended to mean "jacked," as in being stoked or excited. What Jimmy didn't know was that there was a mistranslation. The

Chinese characters on his arms actually meant, "high jacked." Most people never knew and he was never told the true translation.

After Jimmy graduated, he entered the Marine Corp. Recruit Training Depot in San Diego. For the next 13 weeks, he underwent both mental and physical training. For most recruits, the physical training was the most difficult. Recruits endured ten-mile marches, three-mile runs, and lots of calisthenics, including sit-ups and pull-ups. Jimmy had no problem with the exercise part, but he struggled with the classwork. With help from fellow recruits, Jimmy graduated from basic training and was assigned to an aircraft carrier stationed in San Diego. Within six months, Jimmy was in the Middle East supporting the troops in Iraq. His job in the Corp was as an infantryman.

While deployed, Jimmy continued both his vigorous workout regimen and use of dietary supplements. Some of the other marines and navy sailors told him about a new product called Oxy Jack available at the Air Force Base Exchange. Oxy Jack contained caffeine and an amphetamine-like stimulant. Since all armed forces personnel underwent urine drug testing on a quarterly basis, Jimmy was concerned that using Oxy Jack might trigger a positive result for amphetamines. But his service mates told him that they had been taking this supplement for many months and they never failed a drug test. Jimmy started taking Oxy Jack just before his workout in the ship's weight-lifting room. He found that it gave him additional energy, allowing him to work out with more intensity and for longer periods. Soon, he was lifting more weight than he ever did as a civilian.

One day, Jimmy started to experience chest pain that

originated from the sternum and radiated out to his arms. It was very early on a Saturday morning. His ship was docked at Kuwait Harbor, and most of the other sailors and marines were still asleep from Friday night shore leave. A sailor across the gym, who was also working out, heard Jimmy moaning under the bench press. Jimmy started to get up, but then fell forward on his face onto the gym floor mat. His arms didn't move to break his fall. His eyelids were open but his eyes had rolled back into his head. The sailor ran to help Jimmy, but could see that he was having a medical emergency. The sailor rushed to the phone to call the ship's medic, but only got an answering machine. He ran out of the gym and headed for the infirmary. It was 10 minutes before the ship's doctor arrived, by which time Jimmy was pulseless and not breathing. CPR was initiated, including mouth-to-mouth resuscitation and cardiac compressions. A defibrillator was removed from the gym wall, and Jimmy was shocked three times at 300 volts in an attempt to restart his heart. It was all to no avail, and Jimmy Smith was pronounced dead; he was 20 years old.

Jimmy's body was sent to the ship's morgue. There was an extensive investigation as to the circumstances of his death. Where was he the night before? What had he been eating or drinking? Who did he hang out with during his time off? While the investigators could see that he was in excellent physical condition, perhaps there was some congenital vascular malformation that caused his death due to strenuous exercise. When his body arrived back in the U.S., an autopsy was conducted by the Armed Forces Medical Examiner. The external physical exam showed a well-developed and well-nourished male with no evidence of any physical injury. There was a mark on his forehead where he had hit his head when he fell. But there were no bruises or ecchymosis, indicating that blood had stopped circulating to his head when he'd fallen. There were no needle or track marks on his arms or legs. There were no structural or anatomic abnormalities found on his body. All of his organs appeared to be normal except for his heart. There was an 80% blockage in his circumflex artery, one of the arteries that deliver blood to the heart. Each of his other major coronaries was clean, with a minimal amount of atherosclerosis. A toxicology screen was conducted on postmortem blood and urine. The test was negative for all drugs tested by the tox lab. The Medical Examiner concluded that Jimmy died of cardiac arrest induced by an acute heart attack.

*

Jerome Smith, not satisfied that his son died of a heart attack at such a young age, called the California Poison Center because of its excellent reputation and heavy involvement with the toxic effects of supplements. I was the analytical toxicologist on the Poison Center's medical advisory board, and my lab was asked to conduct a more thorough toxicology examination on Jimmy's postmortem body fluids. Jerome appeared more angry than sad about his son's death. I sensed that it might be because it occurred in a non-combat situation and, therefore, in his eyes, this was a loss of a good man. Jimmy's mother on the other hand was devastated.

I requested parts of Jimmy's medical reports prior to his death to see if he'd had any cardiovascular risk factors. At his last physical exam, his total cholesterol was 155, his LDL cholesterol was 92, and his HDL was 65. His blood pressure at the time was 116/82 mmHg. These were all within healthy limits. He also had a normal C-reactive protein. Jimmy was not overweight, had gotten plenty of exercise, and had no history of diabetes or high blood pressure. He was a cigarette smoker, however. I also asked Jerome if anyone in their immediate family had died prematurely of cardiovascular disease, which for men was before the age of 55. He told me no, and that, in fact, both sets of Jimmy's grandparents were still alive in their 80s, and largely healthy. Armed with this information, I went to the National Cholesterol Education Program website and entered Jimmy's data. His 10-year risk score was extremely low at less than 1%. Something outside of the traditional risk factors must have triggered his heart attack.

With this background, I agreed to undergo an investigation of drugs that may have caused his heart attack. Postmortem blood samples were sent to the lab for testing, and used this opportunity to discuss premature heart attacks with my medical students.

"Naturally occurring heart attacks are caused by the rupture of a plaque within a coronary artery," I explained. "This stimulates the formation of a blood clot that blocks blood flow to the heart. But because young people have not time to develop significant plaques within their coronaries, when they have a heart attack it is usually due to vasospasm, which is the sudden narrowing of blood vessels. If this constriction occurs to the extent that it blocks blood flow within one of the coronary arteries, the vessels that deliver blood to the heart itself, an attack can occur. Some people are born with small vessels and are, therefore, at high risk. The autopsy report showed that Jimmy's arteries were of normal size and that he did not have premature atherosclerosis. Having ruled out these possible causes, we next must consider drug abuse, such as with cocaine or amphetamine, as the most likely etiology for his vasospasms. The Armed Forces Toxicology Laboratory, however, had found only a small amount of caffeine but no traces of cocaine or amphetamine in Jimmy's postmortem blood. So we have to look more closely for other drugs that might have been present but not routinely tested for by the military."

Using mass spectrometry, we did find a drug that was not tested by the Armed Forces Toxicology Lab that was present in Jimmy's blood at the time of death. We didn't have a standard at the time to test against, so it took a few days to order the drug and have it tested. When we were sure of what we found, I contacted the family to discuss our results.

"Can you tell us why Jimmy died?" was their first question.

"From the autopsy report, we know that he had an incomplete blockage of one of his coronary arteries," I said. "But this alone should not have caused his heart attack. We did, however, identify a drug that is similar to methamphetamine that may have caused one of his coronary arteries to constrict, reducing blood flow to his heart, causing permanent heart damage."

"I suffered a heart attack a few years ago when I turned 60," Jerome said. "Jimmy was a whole lot younger and was in much better shape than I ever was. What was so different about his attack that caused him to die?"

"It depends on what part of the heart is damaged by the blockage of blood," I explained. "Injury to the regulatory center can interrupt the electrical signals that tell the heart when to beat. An absence of these signals can cause a cardiac arrest. I think this is what happened in your son's case. If someone else had been there, that person could have restarted his heart by electrical shocks. The defibrillator on the wall of the gym was actually used on Jimmy when he was found, but by then it was too late."

"So what is this drug you discovered?" asked Jimmy's mother. "Where did it come from and why was our son taking it?"

"The drug is called dimethylamylamine, or DMAA. It's found in supplements to boost energy for body-building. These supplements are legal and used by many in the armed forces."

"I know that Jimmy was obsessed with building up his muscles," said Jerome.

"Several of Jimmy's friends told us that he was using something called Oxy Jack, which we know contains DMAA," I continued. "In doing research for this case, we learned that other military men have collapsed or died from DMAA."

"What can we do about protecting the other soldiers who are still using this stuff?" Jerome asked.

"I believe that a letter from you and the family members of other victims could be very important in lobbying the U.S. military to remove these products from their commissaries," I said. "The military should also be providing warnings to unsuspecting service personnel. I'll be submitting a report to the FDA about DMAA. A few years back, some investigators from my group were able to petition the FDA to remove ephedra from the market, which is another amine similar to DMAA. You might remember Steve Bechler, who was a pitcher for the Baltimore Orioles. He died after taking three pills containing ephedra. Within one year, the FDA banned that drug. Maybe your son's death can help others from suffering the same fate."

Jerome and his wife felt better that perhaps Jimmy's death would not be without some larger meaning.

*

About the time that I was planning to submit a report to the Department of Defense, it became unnecessary because in late 2011, the U.S. Department of Defense, as a precautionary measure, halted the sale of products containing DMAA from their commissaries. The U.S. Anti-Doping Agency has also banned DMAA-containing products. However, as of this writing, DMAA remains legal. Controlled research studies have not linked DMAA to toxicity if taken at recommended doses. Of course, as with any chemical or drug, excessive use may result in significant medical problems. Moreover, there may be individuals like Jimmy, who have a yet undetermined genetic predisposition to experiencing negative outcomes from ingesting specific drugs. As a result of the Defense Department's removal of DMAA from their shelves, a class action lawsuit was filed in U.S. court claiming false and misleading advertisements against a supplement manufacturer in 2012. While DMAA may eventually be banned, there are many other ephedra-like designer amines that will likely surface, hopefully, without the type of tragic outcome that occurred in the case of Jimmy Smith.

Epilogue

****

An individual may only really know a few thousand people during the course of a lifetime. Casual encounters may increase that number by tenfold or more. A person's influence is much harder to assess. A parent imparts the genetic imprint and fosters an environment that can lead to individual growth; or destruction. A teacher stimulates a generation of thinkers and creators. A preacher is an enabler of inner reflection and spirituality. An entertainer produces relief and an escape from the stresses of the day. A salesman provides the necessities for daily living. A writer allows the mind to imagine. A coach instructs the body to succeed. An attorney finds truth and justice. A lawmaker permits civilizations to evolve. A policeman helps to ensure a civilization's perpetuity. A scientist discovers new pathways for human advancement and comfort. A doctor heals to enable fulfillment of destiny.

Unlike the people in many of these occupations, the contributions made by clinical laboratorians are almost always "behind the scenes." Our names and faces are unknown. We largely don't seek fame or credit for what we do, and we know that none is forthcoming. At parties when someone asks me what I do for a living and I say, "I'm a clinical chemist," it usually requires a long explanation. The alternate response "uh?"

resulting in a polite change of subject or end of the conversation.

Yet when it comes time to make a medical decision about diagnosis, therapy, or patient admission or discharge, our physicians know how important we are. Like the other occupations listed above, our work quietly influences the lives of many. And that is enough gratification for us.

We also provide the answers when it comes to drugs. We can tell you if you've taken too much of a drug or not enough. We can find out what drug you have taken or what you were exposed to and when, even if you don't know yourself or won't admit it. For therapeutics, we can tell you if the prescribed drugs are working or not. Most of all, we can tell you if what you have taken is dangerous or not.

I hope you have enjoyed these cases. This is *Toxicology! Because what you don't know can kill you.*

ABOUT THE AUTHOR

****

Alan H.B. Wu was born in Doylestown Pennsylvania and spent his first years on a farm in New Jersey. In the mid 1950s, he moved with his family first to Chicago and then to Morton Grove, Illinois. He attended Niles West High School in Skokie. Upon graduation, he entered Purdue University, West Lafayette, Indiana, and dual majored in chemistry and biology. Given his interest in clinical chemistry, his advisor Professor Harry Pardue, who was one of the first analytical chemists to train clinical chemists, suggested he attend the University of Illinois, Champaign-Urbana for graduate school. There he received his doctoral degree in Analytical Chemistry from the late Howard Malmstadt, a pioneer in automation for chemistry. Larry Faulkner, former President of the University of Texas in Austin was on his thesis committee. In 1980, Dr. Wu enrolled in the postdoctoral training program in the field of clinical chemistry at Harford Hospital. His mentors were Drs. George Bowers and Robert McComb, renowned for their work on liver enzymes and calcium testing, Robert Burnett, an expert on blood gas analysis, and Robert Moore, who spent his career on clinical chemistry and endocrinology. In 1982, Dr. Wu became Assistant Professor of Pathology and Laboratory Medicine at the University of Texas Health Science Center in Houston, and Associate Clinical

Chemistry Director at Hermann Hospital. After spending 10 years there, he relocated back to Harford Hospital where he became director of the Clinical Chemistry Laboratory, and Professor of Laboratory Medicine at the University of Connecticut, Farmington, and Professor of Pathobiology and Chemistry at the University of Connecticut, Storrs. He left in 2004 to become Professor of Laboratory Medicine at the University of California, San Francisco, and Director of Clinical Chemistry, Toxicology and Pharmacogenomics at San Francisco General Hospital. He is currently a member of the Medical Advisory Board for the California Poison Control Center. Dr. Wu has four children and lives with his wife in Palo Alto California.